The Immunology and Biology of Brain Tumors

The Immunology and Biology of Brain Tumors

Editor

Michael Graner

MDPI • Basel • Beijing • Wuhan • Barcelona • Belgrade • Manchester • Tokyo • Cluj • Tianjin

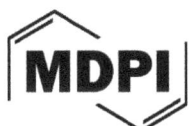

Editor
Michael Graner
University of Colorado Denver
Anschutz Medecal Campus
USA

Editorial Office
MDPI
St. Alban-Anlage 66
4052 Basel, Switzerland

This is a reprint of articles from the Special Issue published online in the open access journal *Journal of Clinical Medicine* (ISSN 2077-0383) (available at: https://www.mdpi.com/journal/jcm/special_issues/immunol_biol_braintumors).

For citation purposes, cite each article independently as indicated on the article page online and as indicated below:

LastName, A.A.; LastName, B.B.; LastName, C.C. Article Title. *Journal Name* **Year**, *Volume Number*, Page Range.

ISBN 978-3-0365-0102-4 (Hbk)
ISBN 978-3-0365-0103-1 (PDF)

© 2021 by the authors. Articles in this book are Open Access and distributed under the Creative Commons Attribution (CC BY) license, which allows users to download, copy and build upon published articles, as long as the author and publisher are properly credited, which ensures maximum dissemination and a wider impact of our publications.

The book as a whole is distributed by MDPI under the terms and conditions of the Creative Commons license CC BY-NC-ND.

Contents

About the Editor vii

Preface to "The Immunology and Biology of Brain Tumors" ix

Martin Voss, AbdulAziz Batarfi, Eike Steidl, Marlies Wagner, Marie-Thérèse Forster, Joachim P. Steinbach, Claus M. Rödel, Jörg Bojunga and Michael W. Ronellenfitsch Adrenal Insufficiency in Patients with Corticosteroid-Refractory Cerebral Radiation Necrosis Treated with Bevacizumab
Reprinted from: *J. Clin. Med.* **2019**, *8*, 1608, doi:10.3390/jcm8101608 1

Jamie D. Costabile, John A. Thompson, Elsa Alaswad and D. Ryan Ormond
Biopsy Confirmed Glioma Recurrence Predicted by Multi-Modal Neuroimaging Metrics
Reprinted from: *J. Clin. Med.* **2019**, *8*, 1287, doi:10.3390/jcm8091287 11

Hao-Yu Chuang, Yu-kai Su, Heng-Wei Liu, Chao-Hsuan Chen, Shao-Chih Chiu, Der-Yang Cho, Shinn-Zong Lin, Yueh-Sheng Chen and Chien-Min Lin
Preclinical Evidence of STAT3 Inhibitor Pacritinib Overcoming Temozolomide Resistance via Downregulating miR-21-Enriched Exosomes from M2 Glioblastoma-Associated Macrophages
Reprinted from: *J. Clin. Med.* **2019**, *8*, 959, doi:10.3390/jcm8070959 23

Mizuto Sato, Ryota Tamura, Haruka Tamura, Taro Mase, Kenzo Kosugi, Yukina Morimoto, Kazunari Yoshida and Masahiro Toda
Analysis of Tumor Angiogenesis and Immune Microenvironment in Non-Functional Pituitary Endocrine Tumors
Reprinted from: *J. Clin. Med.* **2019**, *8*, 695, doi:10.3390/jcm8050695 39

Ryogo Kikuchi, Ryo Ueda, Katsuya Saito, Shunsuke Shibao, Hideaki Nagashima, Ryota Tamura, Yukina Morimoto, Hikaru Sasaki, Shinobu Noji, Yutaka Kawakami, Kazunari Yoshida and Masahiro Toda
A Pilot Study of Vaccine Therapy with Multiple Glioma Oncoantigen/Glioma Angiogenesis-Associated Antigen Peptides for Patients with Recurrent/Progressive High-Grade Glioma
Reprinted from: *J. Clin. Med.* **2019**, *8*, 263, doi:10.3390/jcm8020263 51

Ros Whelan, Eric Prince, Ahmed Gilani and Todd Hankinson
The Inflammatory Milieu of Adamantinomatous Craniopharyngioma and Its Implications for Treatment
Reprinted from: *J. Clin. Med.* **2020**, *9*, 519, doi:10.3390/jcm9020519 63

About the Editor

Michael Graner received his PhD in Biochemistry from the University of Illinois and then completed postdoctoral and research faculty work at the University of Arizona, shifting gears from the Drosophila extracellular matrix to cancer immunotherapy. He then took a faculty position at Duke University's Tisch Brain Tumor Center, followed by his current position as Professor in Neurosurgery at the University of Colorado Denver (Anschutz Medical Campus). He is also a member of the University of Colorado Cancer Center, the Colorado Clinical and Translational Sciences Institute, and the MAVRC Program, and he holds a Visiting Professorship Appointment at the Shenzhen Third People's Hospital (China) and an adjunct faculty appointment at Colorado State University. Graner has a long-standing interest in cell stress responses, which led to cancer vaccine development (including one in clinical trials), which somehow led to the world of extracellular vesicles (EVs). His lab currently concentrates on signaling mechanisms involving EVs, in particular the transfer of stressed phenotypes from stressed tumor cells to unstressed ones via EVs.

Preface to "The Immunology and Biology of Brain Tumors"

Immunotherapy has become a viable treatment modality for a variety of cancers (and referred to as *Science* Magazine's "Breakthrough of the Year" in 2013, as well as ASCO's "Advance of the Year" in both 2016 and 2017). This Special Issue is focused on the relevance of immunobiology in brain tumors, touching on elements of immune suppression, immune stimulation, and the immune microenvironment, with culminations in translational immunotherapy.

Michael Graner
Editor

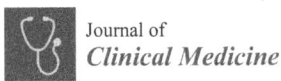

Article

Adrenal Insufficiency in Patients with Corticosteroid-Refractory Cerebral Radiation Necrosis Treated with Bevacizumab

Martin Voss [1,2,3,4,*], AbdulAziz Batarfi [5], Eike Steidl [6], Marlies Wagner [6], Marie-Thérèse Forster [7], Joachim P. Steinbach [1,2,3,4], Claus M. Rödel [8], Jörg Bojunga [9] and Michael W. Ronellenfitsch [1,2,3,4]

1. Dr. Senckenberg Institute of Neurooncology, University Hospital Frankfurt, Goethe University, 60590 Frankfurt am Main, Germany; Joachim.Steinbach@med.uni-frankfurt.de (J.P.S.); M.Ronellenfitsch@gmx.net (M.W.R.)
2. University Cancer Center (UCT) Frankfurt, University Hospital Frankfurt, Goethe University, 60590 Frankfurt am Main, Germany
3. German Cancer Consortium (DKTK), 60590 Frankfurt am Main, Germany
4. Frankfurt Cancer Institute (FCI), University Hospital Frankfurt, Goethe University, 60590 Frankfurt am Main, Germany
5. Department of Neurology, University Hospital Frankfurt, Goethe University, 60590 Frankfurt am Main, Germany; AbdulAziz.Batarfi@kgu.de
6. Institute of Neuroradiology, University Hospital Frankfurt, Goethe University, 60590 Frankfurt am Main, Germany; Eike.Steidl@kgu.de (E.S.); Marlies.Wagner@kgu.de (M.W.)
7. Department of Neurosurgery, University Hospital Frankfurt, Goethe University, 60590 Frankfurt am Main, Germany; Marie-Therese.Forster@kgu.de
8. Department of Radiotherapy and Oncology, University Hospital Frankfurt, Goethe University, 60590 Frankfurt am Main, Germany; ClausMichael.Roedel@kgu.de
9. Department of Internal Medicine 1, University Hospital Frankfurt, Goethe University, 60590 Frankfurt am Main, Germany; Joerg.Bojunga@kgu.de
* Correspondence: martin.voss@kgu.de; Tel.: +49-69-6301-87711; Fax: +49-69-6301-87713

Received: 27 August 2019; Accepted: 27 September 2019; Published: 3 October 2019

Abstract: Cerebral radiation necrosis is a common complication of the radiotherapy of brain tumours that can cause significant mortality. Corticosteroids are the standard of care, but their efficacy is limited and the consequences of long-term steroid therapy are problematic, including the risk of adrenal insufficiency (AI). Off-label treatment with the vascular endothelial growth factor A antibody bevacizumab is highly effective in steroid-resistant radiation necrosis. Both the preservation of neural tissue integrity and the cessation of steroid therapy are key goals of bevacizumab treatment. However, the withdrawal of steroids may be impossible in patients who develop AI. In order to elucidate the frequency of AI in patients with cerebral radiation necrosis after treatment with corticosteroids and bevacizumab, we performed a retrospective study at our institution's brain tumour centre. We obtained data on the tumour histology, age, duration and maximum dose of dexamethasone, radiologic response to bevacizumab, serum cortisol, and the need for hydrocortisone substitution for AI. We identified 17 patients with cerebral radiation necrosis who had received treatment with bevacizumab and had at least one available cortisol analysis. Fifteen patients (88%) had a radiologic response to bevacizumab. Five of the 17 patients (29%) fulfilled criteria for AI and required hormone substitution. Age, duration of dexamethasone treatment, and time since radiation were not statistically associated with the development of AI. In summary, despite the highly effective treatment of cerebral radiation necrosis with bevacizumab, steroids could yet not be discontinued due to the development of AI in roughly one-third of patients. Vigilance to spot the clinical and laboratory signs of AI and appropriate testing and management are, therefore, mandated.

Keywords: adrenal insufficiency; Addison's disease; bevacizumab; cerebral radiation necrosis

1. Introduction

Cerebral radiation necrosis is a frequent complication of current treatment algorithms for malignant brain tumours [1]. Radiotherapy is an integral part of first-line therapy for primary brain tumours like malignant gliomas as well as brain metastases [2,3]. Because the majority of malignant brain tumours are incurable, recurrent disease is almost always inevitable and a second course of radiotherapy can be considered under some circumstances [4], which further increases the risk of cerebral radiation necrosis. Pathophysiologically, cerebral radiation necrosis is characterized by capillary collapse and liquefaction necrosis of brain tissue, which causes an inflammation and vascular endothelial growth factor (VEGF) A-mediated disruption of the blood–brain barrier (BBB) [1,5,6]. Local inflammation can additionally cause necrotic areas to spread and the associated brain edema can greatly exceed the area of BBB disruption. Therefore, cerebral radiation necrosis can cause significant morbidity.

Established therapy for cerebral radiation necrosis is the administration of high-dose corticosteroids [7]. The most commonly employed dexamethasone is a high-potency, long-acting corticosteroid with a biological half-life of 36 to 54 h, which causes profound suppression of the hypothalamus–pituitary–adrenal hormone axis [8]. Patients, especially those on long-term treatment, frequently experience several side effects including weight gain, body edema, skin thinning, striae rubrae, proximal myopathy, steroid-induced diabetes, sleep disturbance, mood changes and sometimes steroid psychosis or depression, osteoporosis, thrombosis, and infections [9]. Bevacizumab is an antibody targeting VEGF-A as a mediator of angiogenesis [10] and established targeted therapeutic approach in some cancer entities including breast and colorectal cancer [11,12]. Much hope was therefore placed in its possible efficacy in glioblastoma (GB). While the first phase II trial of bevacizumab and irinotecan in recurrent glioblastoma with dramatic improvement in MRI presentation (at least a partial response in 63% of patients) sparked enthusiasm [10], three subsequent phase III trials of first-line therapy failed to show any prolongation of overall survival [13–15]. However, similar MRI improvements with reduced gadolinium contrast enhancement had been observed in these studies [13–15], revealing the ability of bevacizumab to reduce the permeability of the BBB without a significant anti-GB effect. As a consequence of the tightening of the BBB, bevacizumab also allowed reducing the corticosteroid doses reported, e.g., in the AVAglio trial (BO21990) [15]. This effect of bevacizumab has been used clinically in small patient collectives as a treatment option for cerebral radiation necrosis [16–18]. However, bevacizumab has not been approved by the European Medicines Agency (EMA) for this indication. Nevertheless, when dexamethasone has to be discontinued as a treatment for patients with cerebral radiation necrosis due to adverse or insufficient antiedematous effects, bevacizumab is an option as part of an individual, off-label therapeutic approach that frequently allows the tapering off of parallel dexamethasone. Since such patients have commonly been treated with dexamethasone for weeks or months, consecutive adrenal insufficiency (AI) has to be considered. The clinical symptoms of AI are nonspecific, and symptoms like lethargy, weakness, and nausea can be misinterpreted as consequences of the tumour treatment or the tumour itself. It may also be challenging to differentiate between AI occurring as a consequence of terminated dexamethasone treatment, which should be substituted with hydrocortisone, and the recurrence of cerebral edema, which is best treated with dexamethasone. In order to evaluate the frequency of AI in brain tumour patients treated with dexamethasone, we chose a collective of bevacizumab-treated patients because corticosteroids can often be terminated and thus basal cortisol can be analysed accurately in this patient collective.

2. Experimental Section

We performed a retrospective analysis of patients treated in our clinic between 2016 and 2019 to identify patients with cerebral radiation necrosis who received bevacizumab and who had at least one documented cortisol value. AI was defined by our laboratory when morning (8–10 a.m.) serum cortisol levels were below 7.25 µg/dL (200 nmol/L) [19]. Cerebral radiation necrosis was diagnosed based on the localization of a lesion within a previously irradiated region, compatible MRI findings including no significant increase in perfusion, non-solid morphology, if available no significantly increased metabolism in O-(2-(18F)fluoroethyl)-L-tyrosine (18F-FET) positron emission tomography (PET) as well as follow-up scans compatible with the diagnosis of radiation necrosis. The patient collective was evaluated with regard to histology, patient age at tumour diagnosis, patient age at cortisol analysis, duration and maximum dose of dexamethasone, the need for hydrocortisone substitution, as well as the radiologic response to bevacizumab treatment. MRI scans including axial fluid-attenuated inversion recovery (FLAIR), T2 weighted, and T1 weighted images before and after application of gadolinium-based contrast agent were analysed by an experienced, board-certified neuroradiologist (M.W.). The extent of edema was estimated on the axial FLAIR or T2 weighted sequence. Response to bevacizumab treatment was defined as a reduction of the edema by at least 25% [18]. Additionally, intracranial contrast-enhancing lesions were measured on postcontrast images as a further marker of the disruption of the blood–brain barrier. Partial response was defined as a reduction of contrast enhancement by at least 50%, and complete response by complete absence of contrast enhancement. Progressive disease was defined as an increase of at least 25%.

Statistical analysis: SPSS Statistics Version 22 was used for statistical analysis (IBM, Armonk, NY, United States). Ethics approval was obtained from the ethics committee of the University Hospital Frankfurt; Goethe University (SNO_01-08). This study was performed in accordance with the declaration of Helsinki.

3. Results

3.1. Successful Treatment of a Patient with Cerebral Radiation Necrosis with Subsequent Adrenal Insufficiency

The therapeutic potential to treat radiation necrosis is exemplified by one patient who had received a second course of radiation for a recurrent glioblastoma. The initial diagnosis was established by tumour resection in 2016. First-line therapy consisted of radiation therapy with a cumulative dose of 60 Gy with concomitant and adjuvant temozolomide according to the EORTC26981 trial protocol [20]. Five months after the end of chemotherapy, a recurrent tumour was diagnosed and resected. Afterwards, the tumour cavity was treated by another course of radiotherapy with a cumulative dose of 20 Gy. The patient subsequently experienced a worsening of headaches and epileptic seizures. An MRI scan showed an increase of contrast enhancing lesions with corresponding edema and led to treatment of the putative radio necrosis with 8 mg dexamethasone daily. In the course of further treatment, parts of the contrast-enhancing lesions were resected in order to differentiate between tumour recurrence and radiation necrosis, and dexamethasone treatment could be ceased. Cortisol had not been analysed at this time point. Histology showed mainly necrosis and scar tissue. A follow-up MRI again showed progressive edema and contrast enhancement, so that dexamethasone treatment was started once again at a dose of 8 mg per day (Figure 1A,B). Despite this treatment, a follow-up MRI again showed progressive contrast enhancement (Figure 1C,D). As a potential side effect of the dexamethasone therapy, the patient became increasingly aggressive towards family members. A 18F-FET PET scan was compatible with radiation necrosis and therapy with bevacizumab was started. After two infusions of bevacizumab, MRI already confirmed a significant reduction of both contrast enhancement and cerebral edema (Figure 1E,F). Treatment with dexamethasone could be stopped shortly thereafter, but serum analysis revealed severe AI with 0.7 µg/dL cortisol. Thus, substitution with hydrocortisone was started. After the therapy with bevacizumab and the end of dexamethasone, the belligerence and rate of epileptic seizures had significantly improved.

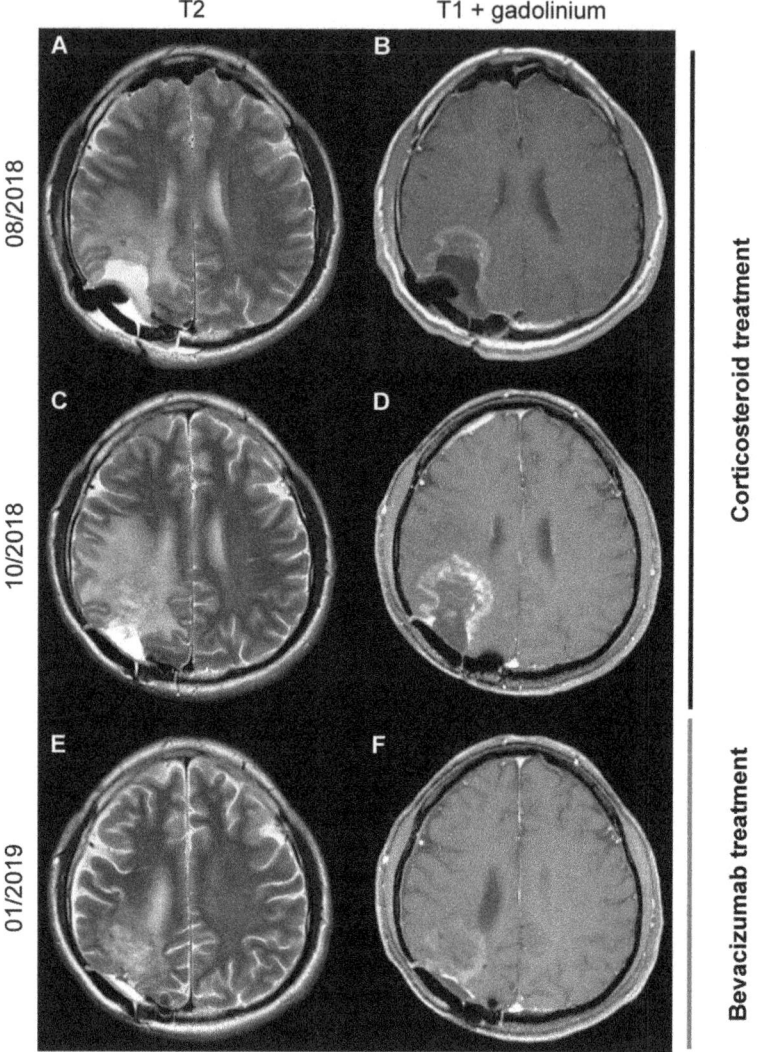

Figure 1. Brain edema and disruption of the blood–brain barrier in an index patient with cerebral radiation necrosis. MRI scans of a 46-year-old patient with glioblastoma of the right parietal lobe (**A,C,E**): T2 weighted images (WI); (**B,D,F**): T1 (WI) after intravenous gadolinium). Re-radiation was applied 10 months before the first MRI. (**A,B**) MRI shows a non-solid, necrotizing lesion with rim enhancement adjacent to the resection defect with surrounding edema. Due to worsening headache and increased rate of epileptic seizures, dexamethasone was started one month later. (**C,D**) the clinical symptoms had declined, yet the MRI shows an increasing extent of the rim-enhancing lesion and of the edema, so therapy with bevacizumab was started one month later. (**E,F**) the first follow-up MRI after two infusions of bevacizumab showed a significant reduction of contrast enhancement and edema. Treatment with dexamethasone could be stopped shortly after, but serum analysis revealed an adrenal insufficiency.

3.2. Identification of a Patient Cohort with Cerebral Radiation NECROSIS and Treatment with Bevacizumab

Forty patients with bevacizumab treatment and cerebral radiation necrosis were identified. Routine cortisol testing is not included in institutional guidelines and at least one cortisol analysis was available in 17 of these patients. Fifteen patients (88%) suffered from primary brain tumours (six GBs, five anaplastic astrocytomas, two diffuse astrocytomas, one ependymoma, one anaplastic meningioma). One patient had a radiation necrosis of the frontal lobe after radiation therapy of a paranasal extracranial tumour, and one patient had a tumour of the cervical myelon without histological confirmation of the tumour entity. Patients' mean age at the time of tumour diagnosis was 43 years (range 20–65), whereas at the time of cortisol analysis patients were 48 years (range 29–67). Six patients were treated with radiation therapy as first-line treatment; 11 patients had repeated radiation treatment of a recurrent tumour prior to bevacizumab. All but two patients were treated with conventional radiation therapy. Radiation doses varied from 54 to 60 Gy for first-line therapy and 20 to 36 Gy for recurrent tumours. One patient treated for meningioma had undergone C12 ion irradiation; another patient suffering from ependymoma had been treated with stereotactic radiosurgery. In three patients, bevacizumab was part of a tumour therapy regimen; the other 14 patients received 1–7 infusions of bevacizumab, specifically as a treatment of radiation necrosis (Table S1).

Bevacizumab was highly effective in reducing local disruption of the BBB and reducing brain edema, as all patients showed a partial response—defined as a reduction of contrast enhancement by at least 50% in the first follow-up MRI. Fifteen of the 17 patients had a reduction of the edema by at least 25%. However, one GB patient 58 years of age receiving treatment for radiation necrosis after re-irradiation with a cumulative dose of 20 Gy suffered a major stroke after seven infusions as a potential bevacizumab side effect. Two patients developed hypertension, which required antihypertensive medication; otherwise, bevacizumab was well tolerated.

3.3. Frequent Adrenal Insufficiency in Patients with Corticosteroid-Refractory Cerebral Radionecrosis

Treatment with dexamethasone was started at a median of four months (range 0–64) after radiation therapy and continued for a median of 141 days (range 18–699). The median maximum dose of dexamethasone was 8 mg (range 4–100), which was reduced stepwise. Dexamethasone was stopped at a median of 61 days after the start of bevacizumab treatment (range −4–372). In 10 patients, the tapering of dexamethasone consisted of a dose reduction to 0.5–1 mg and subsequent switching to hydrocortisone before the analysis of cortisol. In the seven other patients, dexamethasone doses were reduced to either 0.25 mg daily or 0.5 mg every other day, without switching to hydrocortisone. Cortisol analysis revealed an adrenal suppression (<7.25 µg/dL) in five patients (Figure S1). One of these patients presented only a slight reduction of serum cortisol (patient number 5: cortisol 5.7 µg/dL); the other four patients had a marked pathological cortisol value. Additional confirmation of adrenal function via ACTH stimulation was available in 11 patients (two patients with AI and nine patients without AI, as indicated by basal cortisol values) [21]. Notably, the results of all ACTH stimulation tests matched the results of the basal cortisol analysis. Analysis via t-test did not show a significant difference in age, duration of dexamethasone treatment, or time from radiation therapy to start of dexamethasone or to start of bevacizumab between the group of patients with normal adrenal function and the group of patients with AI. The Levene test of variation showed an imbalance of variation for age at cortisol analysis and time from radiation therapy to initiation of dexamethasone/bevacizumab, which could have confounded the results. A comparison of the two groups is given in Table 1. Regression analysis did not show a correlation between cortisol value and duration of dexamethasone treatment or patient age (Figure 2).

Table 1. Comparison of the patients with and without adrenal insufficiency.

	Normal Adrenal Function	Adrenal Insufficiency	p-Values
Number of patients	12	5	
Age at tumour diagnosis (years)	44 ± 15	40 ± 11	$p = 0.587$
Age at cortisol analysis (years)	48 ± 15	48 ± 8	$p = 0.885$
Time from end of radiation therapy to start of dexamethasone (months)	6 ± 8	17 ± 27	$p = 0.397$
Time from end of radiation therapy to start of bevacizumab (months)	9 ± 8	22 ± 28	$p = 0.326$
Duration of dexamethasone treatment (days)	165 ± 132	309 ± 230	$p = 0.120$

Data are displayed as mean ± standard deviation. p-values were calculated using an independent samples t-test.

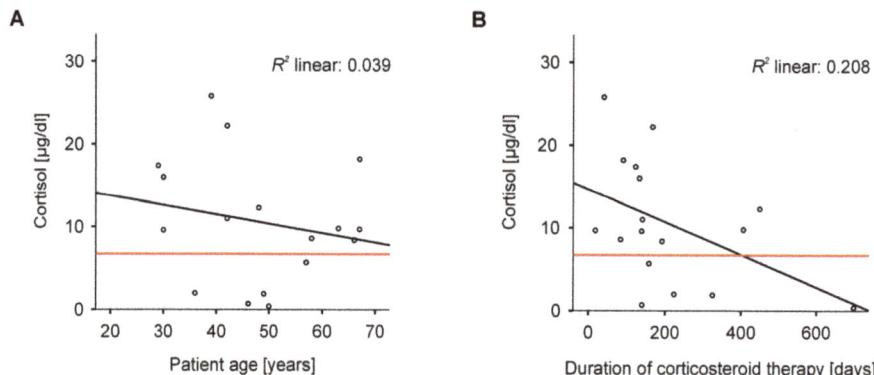

Figure 2. Correlation of cortisol levels with clinical data. Regression analysis of (**A**) patients' serum cortisol level and their age and (**B**) patients' serum cortisol level and duration of dexamethasone treatment did not reveal a significant correlation. The red line indicates the lower limit of the normal value of 7.25 μg/dL (200 nmol/L) cortisol. The linear regression line is shown in black.

4. Discussion

We here report that AI is a frequent condition in patients undergoing bevacizumab treatment for cerebral radiation necrosis, which was detectable in approximately 30% of patients after the cessation of dexamethasone. Our study highlights the need for cortisol testing in brain tumour patients, independently of the treatment duration of corticosteroids.

The frequency of AI in our cohort is in line with a study of patients receiving dexamethasone as a supportive drug for high emetogenic chemotherapy, which revealed a rate of AI of 15% [22]. We further confirm the potent effect of bevacizumab in treating radiation necrosis in our cohort of 17 patients, which has previously been published in a randomized cohort of 14 patients [18]. While severe side effects of bevacizumab have been reported when therapy was administered over longer periods and as part of tumour-targeted treatment regimens with chemotherapy, in short-course and reduced-dose treatment, the side effects profile is most likely significantly less severe [13,18,23].

Almost all patients with intracranial tumours receive dexamethasone during their course of treatment. Dexamethasone is used to treat edema during surgery and radiation therapy and as add-on therapy to chemotherapy to improve the neurological deficit or increase drug compatibility. In patients with recurrent tumours, especially after a second round of radiation therapy, dexamethasone is often required at least temporarily. However, there is increasing evidence for a negative influence of corticosteroids on glioma patients [24]. Dexamethasone-induced leukocytosis is associated with shorter survival and increased risk for lymphopenia [25–27]. Therefore, the lowest possible dose of dexamethasone should always be administered. Nevertheless, balancing dexamethasone doses with edema-associated morbidity can be challenging in daily practice. Patients treated with bevacizumab as part of a chemotherapy regimen or to treat radiation necrosis are the exception in which dexamethasone can frequently be reduced and eventually stopped. Our retrospective analysis revealed a considerable proportion with AI after prior dexamethasone treatment. This is of the utmost clinical importance because AI symptoms can easily be overlooked. Fatigue is one of the most frequent complaints of tumour patients undergoing radiation therapy, but it can also be indicative of AI. We therefore propose testing for AI when terminating dexamethasone treatment with a low threshold, especially in elderly patients and patients who have received dexamethasone over a long period. Additionally, in times of stress (surgery, infection) or unspecified clinical deterioration, cortisol testing should be included in the clinical workup. Notably, none of the patients in our cohort permanently discontinued corticosteroids without prior evidence of sufficient adrenal function. Therefore, specific clinical symptoms of AI were not detected.

The main limitation of our analysis is the small and select sample size, with potential bias for overrating the frequency of AI with regard to the general population of brain tumour patients. Cortisol analysis is not routinely included in the laboratory workup of glioma patients and was only available in 17 of the 40 initially identified patients with bevacizumab treatment for cerebral radiation necrosis (Figure S1). The small sample size may also be the cause of the rather unexpected lack of a significant correlation between the duration of dexamethasone treatment and AI. However, this result is in line with findings in other studies. AI was common in patients with corticosteroid treatment for glomerular disease, but was not predicted by daily dose or duration of treatment [28]. In patients with rheumatoid arthritis treated with corticosteroids, the duration of treatment was also not significantly associated with AI [29].

Another limitation is the bias of a retrospective analysis. It is possible that cortisol was only determined when a higher risk of AI was anticipated and, thus, the proportion of AI may be overestimated. However, cortisol testing is not a common element in routine serum analyses in nonpituitary brain tumour patients, and therefore AI may be greatly underdiagnosed. Further prospective data collection is necessary to estimate the true rate of AI in glioma patients.

Supplementary Materials: The following are available online at http://www.mdpi.com/2077-0383/8/10/1608/s1, Supplementary Table S1. Patient collective. Supplementary Figure S1: Consort diagram of the study population.

Author Contributions: Conceptualization, M.V.; formal analysis, investigation and data curation, M.V., A.B., M.W. and E.S.; writing—original draft preparation, M.V. and M.W.R.; writing—review and editing, M.V., M.W.R., J.B., M.-T.F., C.M.R., J.P.S. and J.B.; visualization, M.V. and M.W.R.

Acknowledgments: The Senckenberg Institute of Neurooncology is supported by the Senckenberg Foundation. M.W.R. has received fellowships from the UCT Frankfurt and funding from the Frankfurt Research Funding (FFF) Clinician Scientists Program.

Conflicts of Interest: J.P.S. has received honoraria for lectures or advisory board participation or consulting or travel grants from Abbvie, Roche, Boehringer, Bristol-Myers Squibb, Medac, Mundipharma, and UCB.

References

1. Miyatake, S.; Nonoguchi, N.; Furuse, M.; Yoritsune, E.; Miyata, T.; Kawabata, S.; Kuroiwa, T. Pathophysiology, Diagnosis, and Treatment of Radiation Necrosis in the Brain. *Neurol. Med. Chir.* **2015**, *55* (Suppl. 1), 50–59. [CrossRef]
2. Weller, M.; van den Bent, M.; Tonn, J.C.; Stupp, R.; Preusser, M.; Cohen-Jonathan-Moyal, E.; Henriksson, R.; Le Rhun, E.; Balana, C.; Chinot, O.; et al. European Association for Neuro-Oncology (EANO) guideline on the diagnosis and treatment of adult astrocytic and oligodendroglial gliomas. *Lancet Oncol.* **2017**, *18*, e315–e329. [CrossRef]
3. Kaley, T.; Nabors, L.B. Management of Central Nervous System Tumors. *J. Natl. Compr. Cancer Netw.* **2019**, *17*, 579–582. [CrossRef]
4. Nieder, C.; Andratschke, N.H.; Grosu, A.L. Re-irradiation for Recurrent Primary Brain Tumors. *Anticancer. Res.* **2016**, *36*, 4985–4995. [CrossRef] [PubMed]

5. Zhuang, H.; Shi, S.; Yuan, Z.; Chang, J.Y. Bevacizumab treatment for radiation brain necrosis: Mechanism, efficacy and issues. *Mol. Cancer* **2019**, *18*, 21. [CrossRef] [PubMed]
6. Duan, C.; Perez-Torres, C.J.; Yuan, L.; Engelbach, J.A.; Beeman, S.C.; Tsien, C.I.; Rich, K.M.; Schmidt, R.E.; Ackerman, J.J.H.; Garbow, J.R. Can anti-vascular endothelial growth factor antibody reverse radiation necrosis? A preclinical investigation. *J. Neurooncol.* **2017**, *133*, 9–16. [CrossRef] [PubMed]
7. Vellayappan, B.; Tan, C.L.; Yong, C.; Khor, L.K.; Koh, W.Y.; Yeo, T.T.; Detsky, J.; Lo, S.; Sahgal, A. Diagnosis and Management of Radiation Necrosis in Patients With Brain Metastases. *Front. Oncol.* **2018**, *8*, 395. [CrossRef]
8. Nicolaides, N.C.; Pavlaki, A.N.; Maria Alexandra, M.A.; Chrousos, G.P. Glucocorticoid Therapy and Adrenal Suppression. In *Endotext*; Feingold, K.R., Anawalt, B., Boyce, A., Chrousos, G., Dungan, K., Grossman, A., Hershman, J.M., Kaltsas, G., Koch, C., Kopp, P., et al., Eds.; MDText.com, Inc.: South Dartmouth, MA, USA, 2000.
9. Roth, P.; Happold, C.; Weller, M. Corticosteroid use in neuro-oncology: An update. *Neurooncol. Pract.* **2015**, *2*, 6–12. [CrossRef]
10. Vredenburgh, J.J.; Desjardins, A.; Herndon, J.E., II; Marcello, J.; Reardon, D.A.; Quinn, J.A.; Rich, J.N.; Sathornsumetee, S.; Gururangan, S.; Sampson, J.; et al. Bevacizumab plus irinotecan in recurrent glioblastoma multiforme. *J. Clin. Oncol.* **2007**, *25*, 4722–4729. [CrossRef] [PubMed]
11. Von Minckwitz, G.; Eidtmann, H.; Rezai, M.; Fasching, P.A.; Tesch, H.; Eggemann, H.; Schrader, I.; Kittel, K.; Hanusch, C.; Kreienberg, R.; et al. Neoadjuvant chemotherapy and bevacizumab for HER2-negative breast cancer. *N. Engl. J. Med.* **2012**, *366*, 299–309. [CrossRef]
12. Hurwitz, H.; Fehrenbacher, L.; Novotny, W.; Cartwright, T.; Hainsworth, J.; Heim, W.; Berlin, J.; Baron, A.; Griffing, S.; Holmgren, E.; et al. Bevacizumab plus irinotecan, fluorouracil, and leucovorin for metastatic colorectal cancer. *N. Engl. J. Med.* **2004**, *350*, 2335–2342. [CrossRef] [PubMed]
13. Gilbert, M.R.; Dignam, J.J.; Armstrong, T.S.; Wefel, J.S.; Blumenthal, D.T.; Vogelbaum, M.A.; Colman, H.; Chakravarti, A.; Pugh, S.; Won, M.; et al. A randomized trial of bevacizumab for newly diagnosed glioblastoma. *N. Engl. J. Med.* **2014**, *370*, 699–708. [CrossRef] [PubMed]
14. Herrlinger, U.; Schafer, N.; Steinbach, J.P.; Weyerbrock, A.; Hau, P.; Goldbrunner, R.; Friedrich, F.; Rohde, V.; Ringel, F.; Schlegel, U.; et al. Bevacizumab Plus Irinotecan Versus Temozolomide in Newly Diagnosed O6-Methylguanine-DNA Methyltransferase Nonmethylated Glioblastoma: The Randomized GLARIUS Trial. *J. Clin. Oncol.* **2016**, *34*, 1611–1619. [CrossRef]
15. Chinot, O.L.; Wick, W.; Mason, W.; Henriksson, R.; Saran, F.; Nishikawa, R.; Carpentier, A.F.; Hoang-Xuan, K.; Kavan, P.; Cernea, D.; et al. Bevacizumab plus radiotherapy-temozolomide for newly diagnosed glioblastoma. *N. Engl. J. Med.* **2014**, *370*, 709–722. [CrossRef] [PubMed]
16. Gonzalez, J.; Kumar, A.J.; Conrad, C.A.; Levin, V.A. Effect of bevacizumab on radiation necrosis of the brain. *Int. J. Radiat. Oncol.* **2007**, *67*, 323–326. [CrossRef]
17. Torcuator, R.; Zuniga, R.; Mohan, Y.S.; Rock, J.; Doyle, T.; Anderson, J.; Gutierrez, J.; Ryu, S.; Jain, R.; Rosenblum, M.; et al. Initial experience with bevacizumab treatment for biopsy confirmed cerebral radiation necrosis. *J. Neurooncol.* **2009**, *94*, 63–68. [CrossRef]
18. Levin, V.A.; Bidaut, L.; Hou, P.; Kumar, A.J.; Wefel, J.S.; Bekele, B.N.; Grewal, J.; Prabhu, S.; Loghin, M.; Gilbert, M.R.; et al. Randomized double-blind placebo-controlled trial of bevacizumab therapy for radiation necrosis of the central nervous system. *Int. J. Radiat. Oncol.* **2011**, *79*, 1487–1495. [CrossRef] [PubMed]
19. Hagg, E.; Asplund, K.; Lithner, F. Value of basal plasma cortisol assays in the assessment of pituitary-adrenal insufficiency. *Clin. Endocrinol.* **1987**, *26*, 221–226. [CrossRef]
20. Stupp, R.; Mason, W.P.; van den Bent, M.J.; Weller, M.; Fisher, B.; Taphoorn, M.J.; Belanger, K.; Brandes, A.A.; Marosi, C.; Bogdahn, U.; et al. Radiotherapy plus concomitant and adjuvant temozolomide for glioblastoma. *N. Engl. J. Med.* **2005**, *352*, 987–996. [CrossRef]
21. Lee, M.T.; Won, J.G.; Lee, T.I.; Yang, H.J.; Lin, H.D.; Tang, K.T. The relationship between morning serum cortisol and the short ACTH test in the evaluation of adrenal insufficiency. *Zhonghua Yi Xue Za Zhi* **2002**, *65*, 580–587.
22. Han, H.S.; Park, J.C.; Park, S.Y.; Lee, K.T.; Bae, S.B.; Kim, H.J.; Kim, S.; Yun, H.J.; Bae, W.K.; Shim, H.J.; et al. A Prospective Multicenter Study Evaluating Secondary Adrenal Suppression after Antiemetic Dexamethasone Therapy in Cancer Patients Receiving Chemotherapy: A Korean South West Oncology Group Study. *Oncologist* **2015**, *20*, 1432–1439. [CrossRef] [PubMed]

23. Wick, W.; Gorlia, T.; Bendszus, M.; Taphoorn, M.; Sahm, F.; Harting, I.; Brandes, A.A.; Taal, W.; Domont, J.; Idbaih, A.; et al. Lomustine and Bevacizumab in Progressive Glioblastoma. *N. Engl. J. Med.* **2017**, *377*, 1954–1963. [CrossRef] [PubMed]
24. Pitter, K.L.; Tamagno, I.; Alikhanyan, K.; Hosni-Ahmed, A.; Pattwell, S.S.; Donnola, S.; Dai, C.; Ozawa, T.; Chang, M.; Chan, T.A.; et al. Corticosteroids compromise survival in glioblastoma. *Brain* **2016**, *139*, 1458–1471. [CrossRef] [PubMed]
25. Shields, L.B.; Shelton, B.J.; Shearer, A.J.; Chen, L.; Sun, D.A.; Parsons, S.; Bourne, T.D.; LaRocca, R.; Spalding, A.C. Dexamethasone administration during definitive radiation and temozolomide renders a poor prognosis in a retrospective analysis of newly diagnosed glioblastoma patients. *Radiat. Oncol.* **2015**, *10*, 222. [CrossRef]
26. Dubinski, D.; Won, S.Y.; Gessler, F.; Quick-Weller, J.; Behmanesh, B.; Bernatz, S.; Forster, M.T.; Franz, K.; Plate, K.H.; Seifert, V.; et al. Dexamethasone-induced leukocytosis is associated with poor survival in newly diagnosed glioblastoma. *J. Neurooncol.* **2018**, *137*, 503–510. [CrossRef] [PubMed]
27. Hui, C.Y.; Rudra, S.; Ma, S.; Campian, J.L.; Huang, J. Impact of overall corticosteroid exposure during chemoradiotherapy on lymphopenia and survival of glioblastoma patients. *J. Neurooncol.* **2019**. [CrossRef] [PubMed]
28. Karangizi, A.H.K.; Al-Shaghana, M.; Logan, S.; Criseno, S.; Webster, R.; Boelaert, K.; Hewins, P.; Harper, L. Glucocorticoid induced adrenal insufficiency is common in steroid treated glomerular diseases—Proposed strategy for screening and management. *BMC Nephrol.* **2019**, *20*, 154. [CrossRef]
29. Joseph, R.M.; Ray, D.W.; Keevil, B.; van Staa, T.P.; Dixon, W.G. Low salivary cortisol levels in patients with rheumatoid arthritis exposed to oral glucocorticoids: A cross-sectional study set within UK electronic health records. *RMD Open* **2018**, *4*, e000700. [CrossRef]

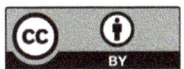

© 2019 by the authors. Licensee MDPI, Basel, Switzerland. This article is an open access article distributed under the terms and conditions of the Creative Commons Attribution (CC BY) license (http://creativecommons.org/licenses/by/4.0/).

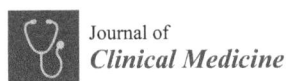

Article

Biopsy Confirmed Glioma Recurrence Predicted by Multi-Modal Neuroimaging Metrics

Jamie D. Costabile [1], John A. Thompson [1,2], Elsa Alaswad [1] and D. Ryan Ormond [1,*]

1. Department of Neurosurgery, University of Colorado School of Medicine, Aurora, CO 80045, USA
2. Department of Neurology, University of Colorado School of Medicine, Aurora, CO 80045, USA
* Correspondence: david.ormond@cuanschutz.edu; Tel.: +1-303-724-2305

Received: 19 July 2019; Accepted: 20 August 2019; Published: 23 August 2019

Abstract: Histopathological verification is currently required to differentiate tumor recurrence from treatment effects related to adjuvant therapy in patients with glioma. To bypass the complications associated with collecting neural tissue samples, non-invasive classification methods are needed to alleviate the burden on patients while providing vital information to clinicians. However, uncertainty remains as to which tissue features on magnetic resonance imaging (MRI) are useful. The primary objective of this study was to quantitatively assess the reliability of combining MRI and diffusion tensor imaging metrics to discriminate between tumor recurrence and treatment effects in histopathologically identified biopsy samples. Additionally, this study investigates the noise adjuvant radiation therapy introduces when discriminating between tissue types. In a sample of 41 biopsy specimens, from a total of 10 patients, we derived region-of-interest samples from MRI data in the ipsilateral hemisphere that encompassed biopsies obtained during resective surgery. This study compares normalized intensity values across histopathology classifications and contralesional volumes reflected across the midline. Radiation makes noninvasive differentiation of abnormal-nontumor tissue to tumor recurrence much more difficult. This is because radiation exhibits opposing behavior on key MRI modalities: specifically, on post-contrast T1, FLAIR, and GFA. While radiation makes noninvasive differentiation of tumor recurrence more difficult, using a novel analysis of combined MRI metrics combined with clinical annotation and histopathological correlation, we observed that it is possible to successfully differentiate tumor tissue from other tissue types. Additional work will be required to expand upon these findings.

Keywords: glioma; diffusion tensor imaging; generalized q-ball imaging; treatment-related effects; multiple resections

1. Introduction

An important challenge facing the neuro-oncological treatment of gliomas is discriminating between tumor recurrence and treatment-related effects using non-invasive diagnostic imaging [1]. Not only do tissue types appear similar on standard magnetic resonance imaging (MRI), but new lesions are often a composite of tumor cells, gliosis, necrosis, inflammatory cells, and neovascularity, which confounds characterization [2]. Moreover, targeted therapies like bevacizumab complicate follow-up imaging even further by modifying vascular endothelial growth factor (VEGF), often causing a "pseudoresponse" with vascular changes resulting in a subsequent decrease in contrast enhancement [3]. Similarly, changes related to radiation or immunotherapy can mimic tumor progression, including changes in T1-weighted (T1w) contrast enhancement and T2-weighted (T2w) hyperintensity, once again complicating imaging-based tissue discrimination [4]. Etiological characterization of lesions observed on longitudinal follow-up scans factors into the clinical decision-making in the course of treatment and prognostic decisions.

While histopathology remains the gold standard for tissue type identification, it is not without its problems, such as the need for additional surgery, sampling bias, and risks of neurological complication [2,5]. Thus, a non-invasive method capable of distinguishing recurrence from treatment effects must be established in order to reduce the dependency on biopsy and improve the efficacy of patient follow-up with noninvasive imaging. Advanced MRI methods such as magnetic resonance (MR) spectroscopy, MR perfusion, positron emission tomography (PET), single photon emission CT (SPECT), diffusion weighted imaging (DWI), and diffusion tensor imaging (DTI) have been used to explore the feasibility of differentiating tumor recurrence and treatment effects with varying success [6–11]. PET-based methods, which measure glucose metabolism, demonstrate some ability in distinguishing glioma recurrence from radiation-induced necrosis. For example, increased fludeoxyglucose (FDG) tracer activity, corresponding to enhanced uptake on post-contrast T1 imaging, is consistent with tumor recurrence, while decreased FDG tracer activity is less specific, typically denoting vasogenic edema, stemming from recurrence and treatment effects [12,13]. Amino acid transport PET-based imaging, especially the use of tyrosine or tryptophan-based tracers, has also been studied to improve the ability to distinguish tumor recurrence from treatment-related changes. O-(2-[18F]fluoroethyl)-L-tyrosine (FET) has been studied since the 1990s and is believed to be more specific for tumor recurrence given the enhanced uptake of glucose in all brain (FDG) versus less amino acids uptake [14]. This should make FET PET more specific than FDG, and there have been a number of cases showing increased uptake of FET in tumors, and it may also be useful at assessing pseudoprogression from true recurrence in glioma [15–20]. However, several other tissue types can also have increased uptake, including brain abscesses, demyelinating processes, epilepsy, and in tissue adjacent to cerebral ischemia or hematomas, making some interpretation of results challenging [14,15,17]. MR perfusion techniques, like dynamic contrast-enhanced (DCE) MRI and dynamic susceptibility contrast (DSC) MRI, yield estimates of relative cerebral blood volume (rCBV) and vascular permeability (k_{trans}), reflecting underlying microvasculature and angiogenesis [21–23]. Studies have indicated MR perfusion's utility in differentiating tumor progression from treatment effects and pseudoprogression [24–26]. However, these techniques are hindered by mixed results [27], model complexity [28], and sensitivity to thresholds [29]. MR spectroscopy, estimating biomarkers like lactate and choline to creatinine ratios, has demonstrated higher diagnostic accuracy than conventional MRI in detecting tumor progression as well, reaching a sensitivity and specificity as high as 91% and 95%, respectively [30]. The diffusion metrics fractional anisotropy (FA) and mean diffusivity (MD) have been useful in differentiating between tissues types as well [31–33]. Recent research on glioblastoma demonstrated that MD can help differentiate between tumor recurrence and radiation-induced necrosis, as it is known that more free water lies within necrotic tissue than enhancing solid tumor [34]. Also, Apparent Diffusion Coefficient (ADC) ratios and mean ADC of tumor recurrence are significantly lower than those of radionecrosis, since higher cellularity (tumor recurrence) contributes to more restricted diffusion [35]. Verma et al. (2013) suggests the combination of low ADC values and high FA values help define the presence of tumor recurrence [2].

High grade gliomas, the most prevalent intracranial neoplasm, are highly heterogenous in the lesion area, have an invasive nature, and often require additional multimodality treatment later in the course of the disease. For these reasons, noninvasive diagnosis, monitoring, and prognosis strategies, such as MRI, must be sought and refined. With the goal to improve the noninvasive diagnostic utility of advanced MRI for gliomas, we studied a group of patients who had imaging localized histopathology. Through the combination of both conventional and advanced MRI modalities, we demonstrate improved efficacy in diagnosing recurrent tumor versus imaging effects related to treatment. These results demonstrate the potential for refining multi-modal MRI assessment of glioma tissue classification, thereby facilitating the clinical decision-making process.

2. Experimental Section

2.1. Patient Information

All procedures and protocols for this study were reviewed and approved by the Colorado Multi-Institutional Review Board (COMIRB 17-1136). Subjects included in this study were patients undergoing repeat resective surgery after radiologically defined tumor progression between August and November 2018 at the University of Colorado Hospital. The patient set consisted of 10 subjects who received prior resection(s) for recurrent glioma with detailed histopathology recorded for 2 or more biopsies (41 biopsies collected in total). Data were collected retrospectively from patient chart review. Two patients received two prior resections; all others received one prior resection. The patient set is divided into two groups: those that underwent radiation therapy prior to repeat resection (RT, $n = 7$) and those that did not (No RT, $n = 3$). For each patient, biopsy samples were collected during surgery from the radiologically-defined tumor region and examined by an expert neuropathologist (B.K.D.). The neuropathologist classified each sample and an expert neurosurgeon (D.R.O.) designated each classification as primarily consisting of abnormal, nontumor tissue (Abnormal), or tumor tissue (Tumor). Patient information is summarized in Table 1.

Table 1. Clinical data of the patient set.

Age	Sex	Location & Pathology	IDH/MGMT/EGFR Status	Time between Imaging and Surgery (Days)	Months Since Prior Resection	RT Prior to Latest Resection	CT prior to Latest Resection	No. of Abnormal Biopsies	No. of Tumor Biopsies
59	M	Right occipital, glioblastoma multiforme	WT/−/lo	2	4.0	Yes	Yes	1	3
34	F	Left frontal, diffuse astrocytoma	MT/NA/NA	2	14.8	No	No	0	4
32	M	Left frontal, anaplastic oligodendroglioma	MT/NA/NA	0	70.4	Yes	Yes	0	4
62	M	Right temporal, glioblastoma multiforme	WT/+/moderate	4	49.2	Yes	Yes	4	1
36	F	Right frontal, glioblastoma multiforme	MT/−/No/BRAF V600E mut	24	27.7	Yes	Yes	6	0
32	M	Right frontal, glioblastoma multiforme	MT/NA/neg	7	62.6	Yes	Yes	0	4
32	F	Right frontal, oligodendroglioma	MT/NA/NA	7	21.5	No	Yes	1	4
58	M	Right tempoparietal, glioblastoma multiforme	WT/+/hi	2	2.8	Yes	Yes	1	2
31	M	Right frontal, diffuse astrocytoma	MT/−/lo	0	51.6	No	No	2	0
42	M	Right frontal, glioblastoma multiforme	WT/NA/lo	10	26.0	Yes	Yes	0	4

Abbreviations: M = male, F = female, MT = mutant, WT = wild type, NA = not available, lo = low expression, hi = high expression, + = methylated, − = unmethylated, IDH = isocitrate dehydrogenase, MGMT = O-6-methylguanine-DNA-methyltransferase, EGFR = epidermal growth factor receptor, BRAF = v-Raf murine sarcoma viral oncogene homolog B, RT = radiation therapy, CT = chemotherapy.

2.2. Imaging Sequence Parameters

All images were obtained using a 3.0-T whole-body MR imager (Signa HDxt; GE Medical Systems, Milwaukee, Wisconsin, USA) between 0–24 days prior to repeat surgical intervention. Acquisition times were 2.5, 5.4, 4.6, 7.8, and 9.0 minutes for non-enhanced T1-weighted (T1w), gadolinium-enhanced T1-weighted (T1ce), T2-weighted (T2w), T2-FLAIR (FLAIR), and diffusion-weighted (DW) images, respectively. For T1w, TE = 2.3 ms, TR = 5.5 ms, and flip angle = 8°. Data were recorded as a 256 × 256 matrix with 1 mm × 1 mm pixel spacing, a slice thickness of 1.2 mm, and zero slice gap. For T1ce, TE = 2.5 ms, TR = 6.8 ms, and flip angle = 8°. Data were recorded as a 512 × 512 matrix with 0.5 mm × 0.5 mm pixel spacing, a slice thickness of 1.2 mm, and zero slice gap. For T2w, TE = 6333 ms,

TR = 80 ms, and flip angle = 142°. Data were recorded as a 512 × 512 matrix with 0.5 mm × 0.5 mm pixel spacing, a slice thickness of 2 mm, and zero slice gap. For FLAIR, TE = 6000 ms, TR = 128 ms, and flip angle = 90°. Data were recorded as a 512 × 512 matrix with 0.5 mm × 0.5 mm pixel spacing, a slice thickness of 1.2 mm, and zero slice gap. For DW images, TE = 85 ms, TR = 16,000 ms, and flip angle = 90°. The diffusion gradient was encoded in 32 directions at b = 1000 s/mm^2 and an additional measurement without the diffusion gradient (b = 0 s/mm^2). DW data were recorded as a 128 × 128 matrix with 0.9375 mm × 0.9375 mm pixel spacing. A total of 50 sections were obtained with a slice thickness of 2.6 mm and zero slice gap.

2.3. Image Processing

Images were processed using a combination of open-source software packages: MRtrix [36], FSL [37], and greedy [38]. Standard MR images (T1w, T1ce, T2w, and FLAIR) were non-linearly registered to the MNI152 (Montreal Neurological Institute, MNI) atlas [39] space using the deformable registration package greedy. Automated tissue-type segmentation was performed on T1w image sets using FSL-FAST (FMRIB's Automated Segmentation Tool) [40]. DT images were preprocessed to remove noise and corrected for distortion and field-bias using MRtrix's dwidenoise [41], dwipreproc [42], and dwibiascorrect [40,43] scripts. After preprocessing, DT images were linearly registered into T1w-space using FSL-FLIRT (FMRIB's Linear Image Registration Tool) [44] and then transformed into MNI-space by applying the affine matrix generated to register the T1w image. Lastly, all image sets were downsampled by a factor of 0.45 with cubic interpolation using MRtrix to avoid oversampling (voxel size: 1.75 mm^3).

2.4. Image Normalization

MR image intensities are acquired in arbitrary units, introducing noise when comparing scans taken at different times. To compensate for artifacts between scans, each MR and DW sequence were normalized across the patient set. Standard MR sequences were normalized using the RAVEL method [45] implemented with the intensity-normalization library [46]. The DW sequence was normalized using MRtrix's dwiintensitynorm.

2.5. Diffusion Feature Space

All diffusion features were calculated using DSI Studio (http://dsi-studio.labsolver.org) on processed and normalized diffusion-weighted images. The diffusion information was reconstructed in two fashions using diffusion tensor [47] and generalized q-space imaging [48]. Diffusion tensor imaging (DTI) determines three primary diffusion directions (and magnitudes) using a tensor, from which the standard diffusion metrics fractional anisotropy (FA) and mean diffusivity (MD) were determined. Generalized q-ball imaging (GQI) is a model-free method that calculates the orientation distribution of the density of diffusing water. Using GQI, the non-standard diffusion metrics quantitative anisotropy (QA) and generalized fractional anisotropy (GFA) were determined. A diffusion sampling length ratio of 1.25 was used. The b-table was checked by an automatic quality control routine to ensure its accuracy [49]. Diffusion feature (FA, MD, QA, and GFA) maps were extracted for each subject from normalized diffusion images.

2.6. Regions of Interest (ROI)

During resective surgery, the locations of biopsies on the patient's MRI were identified using a Medtronic StealthStation S8 Surgical Navigation system (Medtronic, Minneapolis, MN, USA) and application software (Version 1.1.0-39). The biopsy locations were recorded via screenshots. With this information, voxel locations were manually identified on our analytical setup and transformed into MNI-space by applying the patient's transformation affine. A one-half cubic centimeter sphere was used as a facsimile for the biopsy in MR image space.

2.7. Data Analysis

All data analysis was performed using the programming language Python with NiBabel, Numpy, Pandas, Seaborn, Scipy, and Statsmodels modules.

3. Results

3.1. Image Analysis of Biopsy Classifications

The image data analyzed in this study is summarized in Figure 1. Eight MR/DW image features (T1w, T1ce, T2w, FLAIR FA, MD, QA, and GFA) were collected from each patient prior to re-resection. Each image feature was normalized across patients to account for fluctuations in signal acquisition due to environmental and equipment variations (Figure 1A). The image intensities were extracted from ROIs representing the locations of surgical biopsies along with their contralaterally Normal analogs (Figure 1B). Example photomicrographs of the Abnormal and Tumor biopsy classifications from one patient are displayed in Figure 1C.

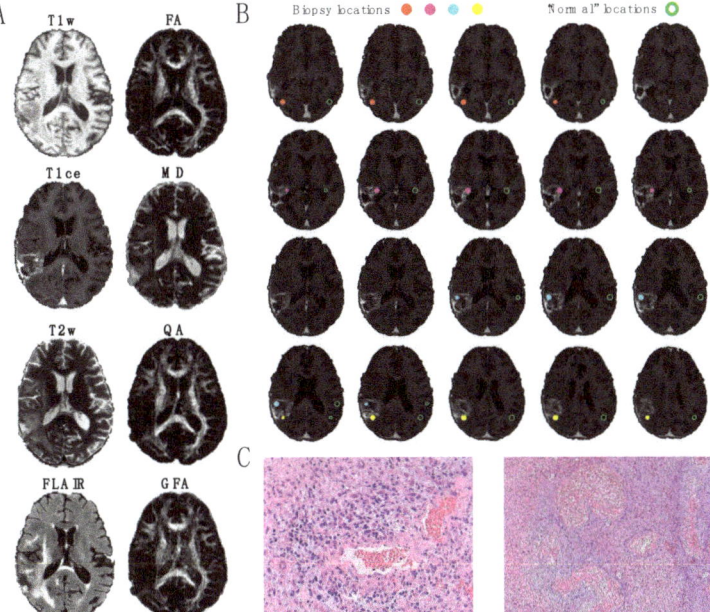

Figure 1. A 59-year old male patient with glioblastoma multiforme. (**A**) Axial slices of the image modalities explored in this study, comprised of four standard MRI metrics (T1w, T1ce, T2w, FLAIR = fluid-attenuated inversion recovery) and four diffusion MRI metrics (fractional anisotropy (FA) and mean diffusivity (MD) quantitative anisotropy (QA) and generalized fractional anisotropy (GFA)). (**B**) Depiction of biopsies from the patient shown in (A). Filled circles indicate the locations of 0.5 mm^3 Regions of Interest (ROIs) representing tissue extractions. Open circles indicate the locations of anatomically similar locations of 0.5 mm^3 ROIs in the normal appearing ("healthy") contralateral hemisphere. For this patient, one biopsy (red) consisted primarily of abnormal tissue and three biopsies (magenta, cyan, and yellow) consisted primarily of tumor tissue. (**C**) Example slides of histopathology used in classification. (Left image) Tumor: Infiltrating high-grade glioma is seen with cytologically pleomorphic nuclei with large areas of necrosis and thick hyalinized blood vessels (20× magnification). (Right image) Abnormal: cortical white matter with extensive gliosis and neuropil vacuolization. Regional necrosis with thick hyalinized blood vessels consistent with radiation necrosis is present (10× magnification).

To explore the effect of radiation therapy on biopsy classification, mean signal intensities were calculated for each ROI and separated based on treatment group (Figure 2). For No RT patients (Figure 2A), differences were detected between Abnormal and Tumor in the T1ce and T2w signals (Tukey's post-hoc test, Family Wise Error Rate (FWER) = 0.05) and between Tumor and Normal in the T1w, T1ce, T2w, FLAIR, FA, and MD signals (Tukey's post-hoc test, FWER = 0.05). No differences were detected between Abnormal and Normal. For RT patients (Figure 2B), fewer image features were deemed statistically different. No differences were detected between Abnormal and Tumor (Tukey's post-hoc test, FWER = 0.05), one difference was detected between Tumor and Normal in the T1ce signal (Tukey's post-hoc test, FWER = 0.05), and two differences were detected between Abnormal and Normal in FLAIR and MD signals. The only difference consistent among treatment groups was between Tumor and Normal for the T1ce image modality; though, the feature demonstrated a reversed behavior between the two groups. Mean Normal signal intensities were equal between groups in all MRI modalities excluding MD (Figure S1).

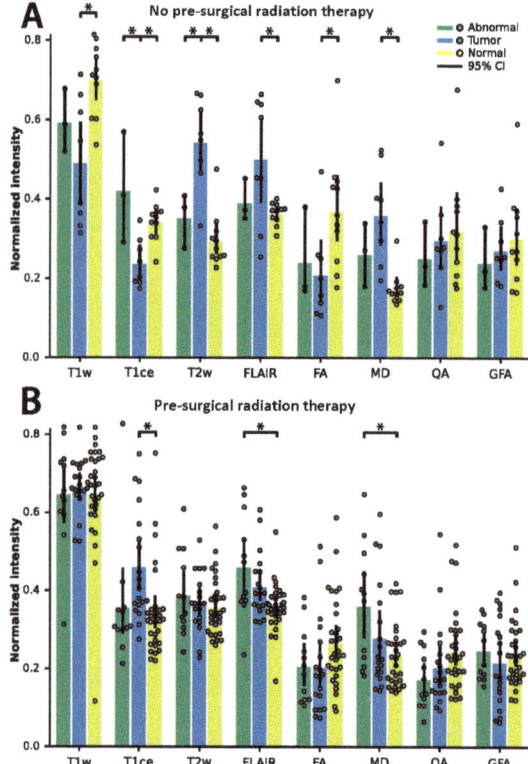

Figure 2. Average ROI normalized image intensity for biopsies classified as Abnormal (green) and Tumor (blue). Contralaterally mirrored ROI locations classified as Normal (yellow). Data separated depending on chemoradiation therapy strategy prior to re-resection: (**A**) patients with adjuvant radiation therapy and (**B**) patients without adjuvant radiation therapy. Error bars show 95% confidence intervals. Asterisks indicate significance determined using Tukey's post-hoc test, $p < 0.05$.

3.2. Logistic Regression Modeling

Given the overall lack of consensus for features that consistently discriminated between treatment groups, we evaluated the ROI image intensities on the voxel-level (Figure 3A,B) to the presence of Tumor (Figure 3C,D) using logistic regression. The regression coefficients provide an estimate of the explained variance each image modality has on the likelihood of the presence of Tumor. Models incorporating all eight image features were created for each treatment and the resulting regression coefficients were calculated (Figure 3C). The significant features consistent in both models were T1ce, FLAIR, QA, and GFA (Student's t test, corrected for multiple comparisons using False Discovery Rate (FDR), $p < 0.05$). However, T1ce, FLAIR, and GFA express inverted information between the models: T1ce shows that for the RT group, higher intensities indicated the presence of Tumor tissue, whereas for the No RT group, higher intensities indicated the presence of Abnormal tissue. The converse is true for FLAIR and GFA: for the RT group, higher intensities indicated the presence of Abnormal tissue, and for the No RT group, higher intensities indicated the presence of Tumor tissue. Therefore, the same approach for differentiating Abnormal and Tumor tissue for patients in the No RT group is not wholly applicable to patients in the RT group (only for QA). Figure 3D illustrates how the No RT and RT models built using the T1ce, FLAIR, QA, and GFA features—perform similarly (area under curve (AUC) = 0.84 and AUC = 0.75, respectively) when accounting for treatment. However, the aggregate model ("All patients", Figure 3D) performed the worst (AUC = 0.60)—showing that the conflicting information (demonstrated in Figures 2 and 3C) degraded the model's ability to differentiate Abnormal and Tumor tissue using multi-modal MRI.

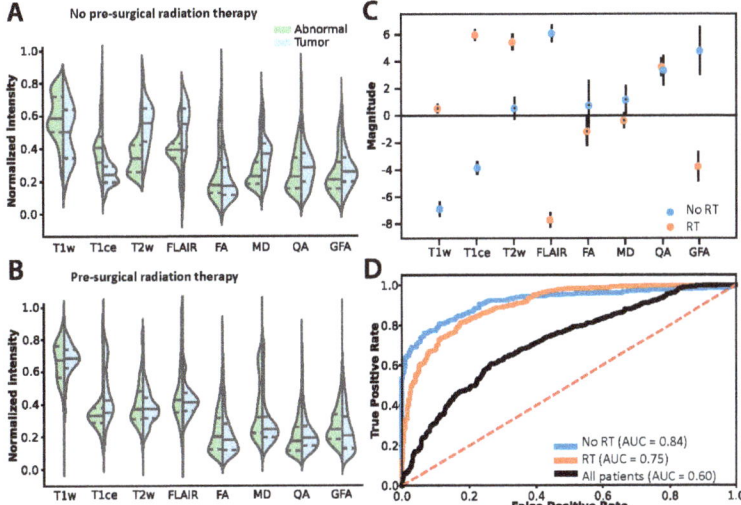

Figure 3. Differentiating the histopathology classifications Abnormal and Tumor on the voxel-level accounting for prior chemoradiation treatment regime. Voxel intensity histograms from the (**A**) No RT and (**B**) RT groups. Solid lines indicate median, dashed lines indicate the lower and upper interquartile interval. (**C**) Logistic regression coefficients: filled circles indicate significant features in the model, open circles indicate non-significant features. Error bars show standard deviation. (**D**) Logistic regression model performance using only the features deemed significant in (**C**). ROC denotes "receiver operator characteristics", AUC denotes "area under curve", and the "All patients" model (built only using features significant in both models) is an aggregate of the treatment groups.

4. Discussion

In order to more specifically evaluate imaging changes consistent with treatment-related effects versus tumor recurrence, we began collecting voxel-based MRI information coupled with location specific blinded histopathological review using a within subject experimental design (i.e., contralesional matched normal voxel as a normal brain control). The goal of this project was to ultimately identify hurdles in predictive modeling regarding imaging diagnoses when longitudinally following patients with glioma after treatment to better assess true recurrence when MR changes occur, incorporating the use of DTI into standard algorithms. Frequently, changes occur on MRI after treatment, which can be difficult to interpret. Treatments such as immunotherapy (still experimental), radiation, or cytotoxic therapy often induce changes in T2w hyperintensity and T1w contrast enhancement that can occur even several years after treatment has ended [4,50–52]. Additionally, targeted therapies, such as bevacizumab, can decrease contrast enhancement and hyperintensity, sometimes masking progression [3]. These challenges in imaging interpretation have been well known for many years. Defining progression in glioma has always been difficult and somewhat controversial.

First described by Macdonald et al., in 1990, the Macdonald criteria were imaging-based criteria to determine glioma progression based on contrast enhancement in two dimensions on CT scans in patients undergoing treatment [53]. This was later adapted to MRI and included four response categories: complete response, partial response, stable disease, or progressive disease. Macdonald criteria is limited by irregularly shaped tumors or nonspecific contrast enhancement from pharmacological treatments, radiation, inflammation, necrosis, pseudoprogression, etc. [54–56]. It also does not account for noncontrast enhancing disease, which is especially important in the evaluation of diffuse low-grade glioma. In 2010, the RANO Criteria consortium published, and later modified, guidelines for the evaluation of treatment response in gliomas and incorporated nonspecific contrast enhancement, multifocal tumors, pseudo-response after treatment, and nonenhancing fluid-attenuated inversion-recovery (FLAIR) hyperintense region in determining treatment response [57,58]. More recent measures of clinical progression have been developed to also help in distinguishing between true progression and pseudoprogression [59,60]. While these measures are important in assessing the global status of the patient and are quite sensitive and specific for global tumor recurrence, they do not answer the challenge of voxel-by-voxel analysis of imaging features specific for tumor recurrence. This study helps to further efforts of predictive, noninvasive modeling by investigating chemoradiation therapy influence on imaging in the process of determining tumor recurrence. These models can also be used to potentially better predict presence of residual disease following surgery, sites of future disease progression, and progression free survival.

This study investigated the effects of surgery alone or surgery plus radiation on voxel-specific pathology. Overall, radiation makes noninvasive differentiation of abnormal-nontumor tissue to tumor recurrence much more difficult. This is because radiation exhibits opposing behavior on key MRI modalities: specifically, on post-contrast T1, FLAIR, and GFA (a GQI feature related to FA). A number of treatment modalities clearly distinguish tumor from abnormal-nontumor postoperatively, however many of these features lose their distinguishing characteristics after radiation (see Figure 2). Specifically, features significant in both models (T1ce, FLAIR, and GFA) demonstrate contrasting information dependent on the postsurgical treatment strategy. T1ce shows that for the RT group, higher intensities indicate the presence of tumor where for the No RT group, higher intensities indicate the presence of abnormal tissue not containing tumor. The converse is true for FLAIR and GFA: for the RT group, higher intensities indicate the presence of abnormal, nontumor tissue, while lower intensities indicate tumor tissue (see Figure 3C). This implies that in order to differentiate abnormal-nontumor tissue from tumor tissue, understanding previous treatment modalities is imperative. The same approach for discriminating one for the other will not work depending on prior treatment.

Violin plots of standard MRI features (Figure 3A,B) help to understand these shifts in a more granular way. Shifts in the histograms happen all along normalized intensity values with nearly all features tested. This is predictable and influenced by treatment strategy, although histograms appear more similar after radiation, demonstrating the difficulty of distinguishing recurrence from post-treatment effects after radiation using standard features of MRI. Standard measurements also differed significantly from normal with or without radiation (Figure 2). However, distinguishing between tumor and abnormal-nontumor was difficult. FA and MD, specifically, provided no information to distinguish tumor from abnormal-nontumor tissue after radiation, although QA and GFA did. Instead, logistic regression helped to illustrate which features contributed most to differentiating the biopsy labels of tumor versus abnormal-nontumor. Hence, the opposing but important findings described previously of T1ce, FLAIR, and GFA and their predictive value in our model. Whereas, QA (quantifies the spin orientation population in a specific direction) remained consistent across treatment models. Ultimately, both models separating images by prior treatment modality (both groups had prior surgery, some with or without chemoradiation prior to re-resection) performed well, while the aggregate model "all patients" performed poorly. This shows that the conflicting information demonstrated in Figure 3C degrades the model's ability to differentiate abnormal-nontumor from tumor tissue on MRI unless separated by treatment modality.

Overall, including non-standard DTI metrics is a useful addition towards differentiation between tumor recurrence and abnormal-nontumor MRI changes, although more is needed in the effort to improve accurate noninvasive prediction of recurrence. This study demonstrates the continued importance of matching imaging data to pathology and clinical annotation to avoid misinterpreting findings on MRI. Ultimately, combining complex datasets including pathology, genomics, epigenetics, imaging, and clinical information will all be important in improving noninvasive assessment of glioma. Future studies including more patients and more precise imaging/pathology correlation will help improve our predictive modeling to the betterment of the care of glioma patients.

5. Conclusions

Radiation makes the noninvasive differentiation of abnormal-nontumor tissue vs tumor recurrence much more difficult. This is because radiation exhibits opposing behavior on key MRI modalities: specifically, on post-contrast T1, FLAIR, and GFA. Ultimately, combining multiple MRI metrics with clinical annotation allows the more successful differentiation of tumor recurrence from other post-treatment effects on MRI.

Supplementary Materials: The following are available online at http://www.mdpi.com/2077-0383/8/9/1287/s1, Figure S1: Comparing average signal intensities from Normal ROIs between treatment groups.

Author Contributions: Conceptualization, J.D.C., J.A.T., and D.R.O.; Data curation, J.D.C. and J.A.T.; Formal analysis, J.D.C.; Funding acquisition, J.D.C., J.A.T., and D.R.O.; Methodology, J.D.C., J.A.T., and D.R.O.; Project administration, J.D.C.; Resources, J.A.T. and D.R.O.; Software, J.D.C.; Supervision, J.A.T.; Visualization, J.D.C.; Writing—original draft, J.D.C., J.A.T., E.A., and D.R.O.; Writing—review & editing, J.D.C., J.A.T., E.A., and D.R.O.

Funding: This research was funded by the Cancer League of Colorado, grant number 183430-DO, and by the American Cancer Society, grant number IRG-16-184-56.

Acknowledgments: We would like to extend our thanks and appreciation to BK Kleinschmidt-DeMasters (B.K.D.) at the University of Colorado, Department of Pathology, for providing detailed histopathological examinations and Lisa Litzenberger for her assistance with the photomicrographs displayed in Figure 1.

Conflicts of Interest: The authors declare no conflicts of interest.

References

1. Bobek-Billewicz, B.; Stasik-Pres, G.; Majchrzak, H.; Zarudzki, L. Differentiation between brain tumor recurrence and radiation injury using perfusion, diffusion-weighted imaging and MR spectroscopy. *Folia Neuropathol.* **2010**, *48*, 81–92. [PubMed]
2. Verma, N.; Cowperthwaite, M.C.; Burnett, M.G.; Markey, M.K. Differentiating tumor recurrence from treatment necrosis: A review of neuro-oncologic imaging strategies. *Neuro Oncol.* **2013**, *15*, 515–534. [CrossRef] [PubMed]
3. O'Brien, B.J.; Colen, R.R. Post-treatment imaging changes in primary brain tumors. *Curr. Oncol. Rep.* **2014**, *16*, 397. [CrossRef] [PubMed]
4. Aquino, D.; Gioppo, A.; Finocchiaro, G.; Bruzzone, M.G.; Cuccarini, V. MRI in Glioma Immunotherapy: Evidence, Pitfalls, and Perspectives. *J. Immunol. Res.* **2017**, *2017*, 5813951. [CrossRef] [PubMed]
5. Costabile, J.D.; Alaswad, E.; D'Souza, S.; Thompson, J.A.; Ormond, D.R. Current Applications of Diffusion Tensor Imaging and Tractography in Intracranial Tumor Resection. *Front. Oncol.* **2019**, *9*, 426. [CrossRef] [PubMed]
6. Matsusue, E.; Fink, J.R.; Rockhill, J.K.; Ogawa, T.; Maravilla, K.R. Distinction between glioma progression and post-radiation change by combined physiologic MR imaging. *Neuroradiology* **2010**, *52*, 297–306. [CrossRef]

7. Galldiks, N.; Stoffels, G.; Filss, C.P.; Piroth, M.D.; Sabel, M.; Ruge, M.I.; Herzog, H.; Shah, N.J.; Fink, G.R.; Coenen, H.H.; et al. Role of O-(2-18F-Fluoroethyl)-L-Tyrosine PET for Differentiation of Local Recurrent Brain Metastasis from Radiation Necrosis. *J. Nucl. Med.* **2012**, *53*, 1367–1374. [CrossRef]
8. Yu, J.; Zheng, J.; Xu, W.; Weng, J.; Gao, L.; Tao, L.; Liang, F.; Zhang, J. Accuracy of 18F-FDOPA Positron Emission Tomography and 18F-FET Positron Emission Tomography for Differentiating Radiation Necrosis from Brain Tumor Recurrence. *World Neurosurg.* **2018**, *114*, e1211–e1224. [CrossRef]
9. Sugahara, T.; Korogi, Y.; Tomiguchi, S.; Shigematsu, Y.; Ikushima, I.; Kira, T.; Liang, L.; Ushio, Y.; Takahashi, M. Posttherapeutic intraaxial brain tumor: The value of perfusion-sensitive contrast-enhanced MR imaging for differentiating tumor recurrence from nonneoplastic contrast-enhancing tissue. *Am. J. Neuroradiol.* **2000**, *21*, 901–909.
10. Barai, S.; Rajkamal; Bandopadhayaya, G.P.; Pant, G.S.; Haloi, A.K.; Malhotra, A.; Dhanpathi, H. Thallium-201 versus Tc99m-glucoheptonate SPECT for evaluation of recurrent brain tumours: A within-subject comparison with pathological correlation. *J. Clin. Neurosci.* **2005**, *12*, 27–31. [CrossRef]
11. Hein, P.A.; Eskey, C.J.; Dunn, J.F.; Hug, E.B. Diffusion-Weighted Imaging in the Follow-up of Treated High-Grade Gliomas: Tumor Recurrence versus Radiation Injury. *Am. J. Neuroradiol.* **2004**, *25*, 201–209. [PubMed]
12. Langleben, D.D.; Segall, G.M. PET in differentiation of recurrent brain tumor from radiation injury. *J. Nucl. Med.* **2000**, *41*, 1861–1867. [PubMed]
13. Ricci, P.E.; Karis, J.P.; Heiserman, J.E.; Fram, E.K.; Bice, A.N.; Drayer, B.P. Differentiating recurrent tumor from radiation necrosis: Time for re-evaluation of positron emission tomography? *AJNR Am. J. Neuroradiol.* **1998**, *19*, 407–413. [PubMed]
14. Wester, H.J.; Herz, M.; Weber, W.; Heiss, P.; Senekowitsch-Schmidtke, R.; Schwaiger, M.; Stöcklin, G. Synthesis and radiopharmacology of O-(2-[18F]fluoroethyl)-L-tyrosine for tumor imaging. *J. Nucl. Med.* **1999**, *40*, 205–212. [PubMed]
15. Floeth, F.W.; Pauleit, D.; Sabel, M.; Reifenberger, G.; Stoffels, G.; Stummer, W.; Rommel, F.; Hamacher, K.; Langen, K.-J. 18F-FET PET differentiation of ring-enhancing brain lesions. *J. Nucl. Med.* **2006**, *47*, 776–782. [PubMed]
16. Hutterer, M.; Nowosielski, M.; Putzer, D.; Jansen, N.L.; Seiz, M.; Schocke, M.; McCoy, M.; Göbel, G.; la Fougère, C.; Virgolini, I.J.; et al. [18F]-fluoro-ethyl-l-tyrosine PET: A valuable diagnostic tool in neuro-oncology, but not all that glitters is glioma. *Neuro Oncol.* **2013**, *15*, 341–351. [CrossRef] [PubMed]
17. Hutterer, M.; Ebner, Y.; Riemenschneider, M.J.; Willuweit, A.; McCoy, M.; Egger, B.; Schröder, M.; Wendl, C.; Hellwig, D.; Grosse, J.; et al. Epileptic Activity Increases Cerebral Amino Acid Transport Assessed by 18F-Fluoroethyl-l-Tyrosine Amino Acid PET: A Potential Brain Tumor Mimic. *J. Nucl. Med.* **2017**, *58*, 129–137. [CrossRef]
18. Pichler, R.; Dunzinger, A.; Wurm, G.; Pichler, J.; Weis, S.; Nussbaumer, K.; Topakian, R.; Aigner, R.M. Is there a place for FET PET in the initial evaluation of brain lesions with unknown significance? *Eur. J. Nucl. Med. Mol. Imaging* **2010**, *37*, 1521–1528. [CrossRef]
19. Kebir, S.; Fimmers, R.; Galldiks, N.; Schäfer, N.; Mack, F.; Schaub, C.; Stuplich, M.; Niessen, M.; Tzaridis, T.; Simon, M.; et al. Late Pseudoprogression in Glioblastoma: Diagnostic Value of Dynamic O-(2-[18F]fluoroethyl)-L-Tyrosine PET. *Clin. Cancer Res.* **2016**, *22*, 2190–2196. [CrossRef]
20. Galldiks, N.; Dunkl, V.; Stoffels, G.; Hutterer, M.; Rapp, M.; Sabel, M.; Reifenberger, G.; Kebir, S.; Dorn, F.; Blau, T.; et al. Diagnosis of pseudoprogression in patients with glioblastoma using O-(2-[18F]fluoroethyl)-l-tyrosine PET. *Eur. J. Nucl. Med. Mol. Imaging* **2015**, *42*, 685–695. [CrossRef]
21. Cha, S.; Knopp, E.A.; Johnson, G.; Wetzel, S.G.; Litt, A.W.; Zagzag, D. Intracranial Mass Lesions: Dynamic Contrast-enhanced Susceptibility-weighted Echo-planar Perfusion MR Imaging. *Radiology* **2002**, *223*, 11–29. [CrossRef] [PubMed]
22. Narang, J.; Jain, R.; Arbab, A.S.; Mikkelsen, T.; Scarpace, L.; Rosenblum, M.L.; Hearshen, D.; Babajani-Feremi, A. Differentiating treatment-induced necrosis from recurrent/progressive brain tumor using nonmodel-based semiquantitative indices derived from dynamic contrast-enhanced T1-weighted MR perfusion. *Neuro Oncol.* **2011**, *13*, 1037–1046. [CrossRef] [PubMed]
23. Ahmed, R.; Oborski, M.J.; Hwang, M.; Lieberman, F.S.; Mountz, J.M. Malignant gliomas: Current perspectives in diagnosis, treatment, and early response assessment using advanced quantitative imaging methods. *Cancer Manag. Res.* **2014**, *6*, 149–170. [PubMed]

24. Bisdas, S.; Naegele, T.; Ritz, R.; Dimostheni, A.; Pfannenberg, C.; Reimold, M.; Koh, T.S.; Ernemann, U. Distinguishing Recurrent High-grade Gliomas from Radiation Injury. A Pilot Study Using Dynamic Contrast-enhanced MR Imaging. *Acad. Radiol.* **2011**, *18*, 575–583. [CrossRef] [PubMed]
25. Hazle, J.D.; Jackson, E.F.; Schomer, D.F.; Leeds, N.E. Dynamic imaging of intracranial lesions using fast spin-echo imaging: Differentiation of brain tumors and treatment effects. *J. Magn. Reson. Imaging* **1997**, *7*, 1084–1093. [CrossRef] [PubMed]
26. Aronen, H.J.; Perkiö, J. Dynamic susceptibility contrast MRI of gliomas. *Neuroimaging Clin. N. Am.* **2002**, *12*, 501–523. [CrossRef]
27. Jain, R.K.; Tong, R.T.; Munn, L.L. Effect of vascular normalization by antiangiogenic therapy on interstitial hypertension, peritumor edema, and lymphatic metastasis: Insights from a mathematical model. *Cancer Res.* **2007**, *67*, 2729–2735. [CrossRef] [PubMed]
28. Buckley, D.L. Uncertainty in the analysis of tracer kinetics using dynamic contrast enhanced T1-weighted MRI. *Magn. Reson. Med.* **2002**, *47*, 601–606. [CrossRef]
29. Kruser, T.J.; Mehta, M.P.; Robins, H.I. Pseudoprogression after glioma therapy: A comprehensive review. *Expert Rev. Neurother.* **2013**, *13*, 389–403. [CrossRef]
30. Van Dijken, B.R.J.; van Laar, P.J.; Holtman, G.A.; van der Hoorn, A. Diagnostic accuracy of magnetic resonance imaging techniques for treatment response evaluation in patients with high-grade glioma, a systematic review and meta-analysis. *Eur. Radiol.* **2017**, *27*, 4129–4144. [CrossRef]
31. Wang, S.; Kim, S.; Chawla, S.; Wolf, R.L.; Zhang, W.G.; O'Rourke, D.M.; Judy, K.D.; Melhem, E.R.; Poptani, H. Differentiation between glioblastomas and solitary brain metastases using diffusion tensor imaging. *NeuroImage* **2009**, *44*, 653–660. [CrossRef] [PubMed]
32. Li, Y.; Zhang, W. Quantitative evaluation of diffusion tensor imaging for clinical management of glioma. *Neurosurg. Rev.* **2018**, 1–11. [CrossRef] [PubMed]
33. Sundgren, P.C.; Fan, X.; Weybright, P.; Welsh, R.C.; Carlos, R.C.; Petrou, M.; McKeever, P.E.; Chenevert, T.L. Differentiation of recurrent brain tumor versus radiation injury using diffusion tensor imaging in patients with new contrast-enhancing lesions. *Magn. Reson. Imaging* **2006**, *24*, 1131–1142. [CrossRef] [PubMed]
34. Sinha, S.; Bastin, M.E.; Whittle, I.R.; Wardlaw, J.M. Diffusion tensor MR imaging of high-grade cerebral gliomas. *Am. J. Neuroradiol.* **2002**, *23*, 520–527. [PubMed]
35. Xu, J.L.; Li, Y.L.; Lian, J.M.; Dou, S.W.; Yan, F.S.; Wu, H.; Shi, D.P. Distinction between postoperative recurrent glioma and radiation injury using MR diffusion tensor imaging. *Neuroradiology* **2010**, *52*, 1193–1199. [CrossRef]
36. Tournier, J.D.; Calamante, F.; Connelly, A. MRtrix: Diffusion tractography in crossing fiber regions. *Int. J. Imaging Syst. Technol.* **2012**, *22*, 53–66. [CrossRef]
37. Jenkinson, M.; Beckmann, C.F.; Behrens, T.E.J.; Woolrich, M.W.; Smith, S.M. FSL. *NeuroImage* **2012**, *62*, 782–790. [CrossRef]
38. Joshi, S.; Davis, B.; Jomier, M.; Gerig, G. Unbiased diffeomorphic atlas construction for computational anatomy. *NeuroImage* **2004**, *23*, S151–S160. [CrossRef]
39. Fonov, V.; Evans, A.C.; Botteron, K.; Almli, C.R.; McKinstry, R.C.; Collins, D.L. Unbiased average age-appropriate atlases for pediatric studies. *NeuroImage* **2011**, *54*, 313–327. [CrossRef]
40. Zhang, Y.; Brady, M.; Smith, S. Segmentation of brain MR images through a hidden Markov random field model and the expectation-maximization algorithm. *IEEE Trans. Med. Imaging* **2001**, *20*, 45–57. [CrossRef]
41. Veraart, J.; Novikov, D.S.; Christiaens, D.; Ades-aron, B.; Sijbers, J.; Fieremans, E. Denoising of diffusion MRI using random matrix theory. *NeuroImage* **2016**, *142*, 394–406. [CrossRef] [PubMed]
42. Andersson, J.L.R.; Sotiropoulos, S.N. An integrated approach to correction for off-resonance effects and subject movement in diffusion MR imaging. *NeuroImage* **2016**, *125*, 1063–1078. [CrossRef] [PubMed]
43. Smith, S.M.; Jenkinson, M.; Woolrich, M.W.; Beckmann, C.F.; Behrens, T.E.J.; Johansen-Berg, H.; Bannister, P.R.; De Luca, M.; Drobnjak, I.; Flitney, D.E.; et al. Advances in functional and structural MR image analysis and implementation as FSL. *NeuroImage* **2004**, *23* (Suppl. S1), S208–S219. [CrossRef]
44. Jenkinson, M.; Bannister, P.; Brady, M.; Smith, S. Improved optimization for the robust and accurate linear registration and motion correction of brain images. *NeuroImage* **2002**, *17*, 825–841. [CrossRef] [PubMed]
45. Fortin, J.-P.; Sweeney, E.M.; Muschelli, J.; Crainiceanu, C.M.; Shinohara, R.T. Alzheimer's Disease Neuroimaging Initiative Removing inter-subject technical variability in magnetic resonance imaging studies. *NeuroImage* **2016**, *132*, 198–212. [CrossRef] [PubMed]

46. Reinhold, J.C.; Dewey, B.E.; Carass, A.; Prince, J.L. Evaluating the impact of intensity normalization on MR image synthesis. In Proceedings of the Medical Imaging 2019: Image Processing, San Diego, CA, USA, 19–21 February 2019; Angelini, E.D., Landman, B.A., Eds.; SPIE: Bellingham, DC, USA, 2019; Volume 10949, p. 126.
47. Basser, P.J.; Mattiello, J.; LeBihan, D. MR diffusion tensor spectroscopy and imaging. *Biophys. J.* **1994**, *66*, 259–267. [CrossRef]
48. Yeh, F.C.; Wedeen, V.J.; Tseng, W.Y.I. Generalized q-sampling imaging. *IEEE Trans. Med. Imaging* **2010**, *29*, 1626–1635. [PubMed]
49. Schilling, K.G.; Yeh, F.-C.; Nath, V.; Hansen, C.; Williams, O.; Resnick, S.; Anderson, A.W.; Landman, B.A. A fiber coherence index for quality control of B-table orientation in diffusion MRI scans. *Magn. Reson. Imaging* **2019**, *58*, 82–89. [CrossRef] [PubMed]
50. Roldán, G.B.; Scott, J.N.; McIntyre, J.B.; Dharmawardene, M.; de Robles, P.A.; Magliocco, A.M.; Yan, E.S.Y.; Parney, I.F.; Forsyth, P.A.; Cairncross, J.G.; et al. Population-based study of pseudoprogression after chemoradiotherapy in GBM. *Can. J. Neurol. Sci.* **2009**, *36*, 617–622. [CrossRef] [PubMed]
51. Sanghera, P.; Perry, J.; Sahgal, A.; Symons, S.; Aviv, R.; Morrison, M.; Lam, K.; Davey, P.; Tsao, M.N. Pseudoprogression following chemoradiotherapy for glioblastoma multiforme. *Can. J. Neurol. Sci.* **2010**, *37*, 36–42. [CrossRef] [PubMed]
52. Linhares, P.; Carvalho, B.; Figueiredo, R.; Reis, R.M.; Vaz, R. Early Pseudoprogression following Chemoradiotherapy in Glioblastoma Patients: The Value of RANO Evaluation. *J. Oncol.* **2013**, *2013*, 690585. [CrossRef] [PubMed]
53. Macdonald, D.R.; Cascino, T.L.; Schold, S.C.; Cairncross, J.G. Response criteria for phase II studies of supratentorial malignant glioma. *J. Clin. Oncol.* **1990**, *8*, 1277–1280. [CrossRef] [PubMed]
54. De Wit, M.C.Y.; De Bruin, H.G.; Eijkenboom, W.; Sillevis Smitt, P.A.E.; Van Den Bent, M.J. Immediate post-radiotherapy changes in malignant glioma can mimic tumor progression. *Neurology* **2004**, *63*, 535–537. [CrossRef] [PubMed]
55. Van den Bent, M.J.; Vogelbaum, M.A.; Wen, P.Y.; Macdonald, D.R.; Chang, S.M. End Point Assessment in Gliomas: Novel Treatments Limit Usefulness of Classical Macdonald's Criteria. *J. Clin. Oncol.* **2009**, *27*, 2905–2908. [CrossRef] [PubMed]
56. Sorensen, A.G.; Batchelor, T.T.; Wen, P.Y.; Zhang, W.T.; Jain, R.K. Response criteria for glioma. *Nat. Clin. Pract. Oncol.* **2008**, *5*, 634–644. [CrossRef] [PubMed]
57. Wen, P.Y.; Macdonald, D.R.; Reardon, D.A.; Cloughesy, T.F.; Sorensen, A.G.; Galanis, E.; DeGroot, J.; Wick, W.; Gilbert, M.R.; Lassman, A.B.; et al. Updated response assessment criteria for high-grade gliomas: Response assessment in neuro-oncology working group. *J. Clin. Oncol.* **2010**, *28*, 1963–1972. [CrossRef] [PubMed]
58. Vogelbaum, M.A.; Jost, S.; Aghi, M.K.; Heimberger, A.B.; Sampson, J.H.; Wen, P.Y.; Macdonald, D.R.; Van den Bent, M.J.; Chang, S.M. Application of novel response/progression measures for surgically delivered therapies for gliomas: Response Assessment in Neuro-Oncology (RANO) Working Group. *Neurosurgery* **2012**, *70*, 234–243. [CrossRef] [PubMed]
59. Nayak, L.; DeAngelis, L.M.; Brandes, A.A.; Peereboom, D.M.; Galanis, E.; Lin, N.U.; Soffietti, R.; Macdonald, D.R.; Chamberlain, M.; Perry, J.; et al. The Neurologic Assessment in Neuro-Oncology (NANO) scale: A tool to assess neurologic function for integration into the Response Assessment in Neuro-Oncology (RANO) criteria. *Neuro Oncol.* **2017**, *19*, 625–635. [CrossRef] [PubMed]
60. Ung, T.H.; Ney, D.E.; Damek, D.; Rusthoven, C.G.; Youssef, A.S.; Lillehei, K.O.; Ormond, D.R. The Neurologic Assessment in Neuro-Oncology (NANO) Scale as an Assessment Tool for Survival in Patients With Primary Glioblastoma. *Neurosurgery* **2019**, *84*, 687–695. [CrossRef]

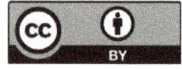

© 2019 by the authors. Licensee MDPI, Basel, Switzerland. This article is an open access article distributed under the terms and conditions of the Creative Commons Attribution (CC BY) license (http://creativecommons.org/licenses/by/4.0/).

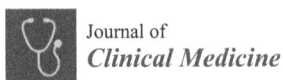

Article

Preclinical Evidence of STAT3 Inhibitor Pacritinib Overcoming Temozolomide Resistance via Downregulating miR-21-Enriched Exosomes from M2 Glioblastoma-Associated Macrophages

Hao-Yu Chuang [1,2,3], Yu-kai Su [4,5,6,7], Heng-Wei Liu [4,5,6,7], Chao-Hsuan Chen [8,9,10,11], Shao-Chih Chiu [8,9,10,11], Der-Yang Cho [8,9,10,11], Shinn-Zong Lin [12,13], Yueh-Sheng Chen [14,*] and Chien-Min Lin [5,6,7,*]

1. Graduate Institute of Clinical Medical Science, China Medical University, Taichung 404, Taiwan
2. Department of Neurosurgery, An Nan Hospital, China Medical University, Tainan 709, Taiwan
3. Department of Neurosurgery, China Medical University Beigang Hospital, Yunlin 651, Taiwan
4. Graduate Institute of Clinical Medicine, College of Medicine, Taipei Medical University, Taipei City 11031, Taiwan
5. Department of Neurology, School of Medicine, College of Medicine, Taipei Medical University, Taipei City 11031, Taiwan
6. Division of Neurosurgery, Department of Surgery, Taipei Medical University-Shuang Ho Hospital, New Taipei City 23561, Taiwan
7. Taipei Neuroscience Institute, Taipei Medical University, Taipei 11031, Taiwan
8. Center for Cell Therapy, China Medical University Hospital, Taichung 404, Taiwan
9. Drug Development Center, China Medical University, Taichung 404, Taiwan
10. Graduate Institute of Biomedical Sciences, China Medical University, Taichung 404, Taiwan
11. Department of Neurosurgery, China Medical University Hospital, Taichung 404, Taiwan
12. Bioinnovation Center, Buddhist Tzu Chi Medical Foundation, Hualien 97004, Taiwan
13. Department of Neurosurgery, Tzu Chi University, Hualien Tzu Chi Hospital, Buddhist Tzu Chi Medical Foundation, Hualien 97004, Taiwan
14. Department of Biomedical Imaging and Radiological Science, China Medical University, Taichung 404, Taiwan
* Correspondence: yuehsc@mail.cmu.edu.tw (Y.-S.C.); m513092004@tmu.edu.tw (C.-M.L.); Tel.: +886-2-2490088 (ext. 8881) (Y.-S.C.); +886-2-2490088 (ext. 8885) (C.-M.L.); Fax: +886-2-2248-0900 (Y.-S.C. & C.-M.L.)

Received: 30 May 2019; Accepted: 29 June 2019; Published: 2 July 2019

Abstract: Background: The tumor microenvironment (TME) plays a crucial role in virtually every aspect of tumorigenesis of glioblastoma multiforme (GBM). A dysfunctional TME promotes drug resistance, disease recurrence, and distant metastasis. Recent evidence indicates that exosomes released by stromal cells within the TME may promote oncogenic phenotypes via transferring signaling molecules such as cytokines, proteins, and microRNAs. Results: In this study, clinical GBM samples were collected and analyzed. We found that GBM-associated macrophages (GAMs) secreted exosomes which were enriched with oncomiR-21. Coculture of GAMs (and GAM-derived exosomes) and GBM cell lines increased GBM cells' resistance against temozolomide (TMZ) by upregulating the prosurvival gene programmed cell death protein 4 (PDCD4) and stemness markers SRY (sex determining region y)-box 2 (Sox2), signal transducer and activator of transcription 3 (STAT3), Nestin, and miR-21-5p and increasing the M2 cytokines interleukin 6 (IL-6) and transforming growth factor beta 1(TGF-β1) secreted by GBM cells, promoting the M2 polarization of GAMs. Subsequently, pacritinib treatment suppressed GBM tumorigenesis and stemness; more importantly, pacritinib-treated GBM cells showed a markedly reduced ability to secret M2 cytokines and reduced miR-21-enriched exosomes secreted by GAMs. Pacritinib-mediated effects were accompanied by a reduction of oncomiR miR-21-5p, by which the tumor suppressor PDCD4 was targeted. We subsequently established patient-derived xenograft (PDX) models where mice bore patient GBM and GAMs. Treatment with pacritinib and the combination of pacritinib and TMZ appeared to significantly reduce the tumorigenesis of GBM/GAM PDX mice as well as overcome TMZ resistance and M2 polarization of GAMs. Conclusion: In summation, we showed the potential of pacritinib alone or in combination with TMZ to suppress GBM tumorigenesis via modulating STAT3/miR-21/PDCD4 signaling. Further investigations are warranted for adopting pacritinib for the treatment of TMZ-resistant GBM in clinical settings.

Keywords: tumor microenvironment (TME); glioblastoma multiforme (GBM); ; GBM-associated macrophages (GAMs); exosomes; oncomiR-21; STAT3 inhibitor

1. Introduction

Glioblastoma multiforme (GBM) is the most aggressive brain tumor of glial origin and has a poor median survival of 14 months [1]. One of the reasons for its malignancy and challenging therapeutics development lies in its heterogeneous nature at the cellular and molecular levels. It is now generally recognized that GBM is composed of a subpopulation of glioma stem cells (GSCs), capable of tumor initiation and progressive self-renewal upon treatments, and other cells within the tumor microenvironment (TME). The TME contains cancerous cells surrounded by parenchymal cells, including endothelial/vascular cells, microglia, and immune cells [2]. One of the major cell types from the GBM TME is glioblastoma-associated macrophages (GAMs). GAMs have been shown to contribute to the progression of GBM. For instance, the presence of M2 GAMs has been shown to promote the growth and metastasis of GBM cells [2,3].

More importantly, emerging evidence indicates the dynamic intercellular communications within the GBM TME via secretions of cytokines, chemicals, and signaling molecules. Among these, secreted exosomes represent a class of small bilayered particles (ranging from 50 to 150 nm in diameter) which have been extensively explored for their roles in GBM tumorigenesis over the past few years [4]. Recent studies have shed light on the diverse functions of exosomes involved in GBM tumorigenesis. For instance, exosomes released from human GBM cell lines contain various types of heat shock proteins and transforming growth factor beta 1(TGF-β1) which are proposed to exert immune suppressive roles in GBM [5]. In addition, serum-derived exosomes from GBM patients and Cerebrospinal fluid (CSF) derived exosomes were shown to contain a high level of miR-221, serving as a potential GBM biomarker [6]. A recent study demonstrated that microglia also communicate and affect the function of glioma via the release of exosomes [7]. These findings suggest that there is a potential area for therapeutics development via interrupting the intracellular communications between GBM cells and their TME by means of exosomes. However, the role of exosomes derived from M2 GAMs has not been fully appreciated.

In this study, we first demonstrated that when human GBM cell lines were cocultured with clinically isolated glioblastoma-associated macrophages, this significantly enhanced colony formation ability and tumor sphere generation in association with an increased expression of Sox2, STAT3, interleukin 6 (IL-6), and Nestin and a decrease in glial fibrillary acidic protein (GFAP). Subsequently, exosomes released into the culture medium of GAMs were isolated and cocultured with GBM cell lines. A similarly increased tumorigenic property was observed in addition to the increased resistance against temozolomide (TMZ). More importantly, miR-21, a oncomiR, was identified as the most abundant microRNA species in the exosomes released from the GAMs. We then provided evidence for the positive association between miR-21 level and GBM malignancy. Exogenously increased miR-21 in GBM cells increased their ability to polarize GAMs towards the M2 phenotype, and the reduction of miR-21 reversed these properties. In addition, we showed that miR-21-mediated oncogenic properties were associated with their targeting/inhibitory function on PDCD4 (a tumor suppressor). An increased miR-21 level in the GBM cells led to their increased ability to polarize GAMs towards the M2 phenotype by the increased secretion of the M2 cytokines IL-6 and TGF-β1.

Subsequently, we examined the feasibility of applying pacritinib, an inhibitor of the STAT3-associated pathway, as an anti-GBM agent. We showed that pacritinib treatment significantly reduced cell viability and colony/tumor sphere formation in association with reduced levels of STAT3, Sox2, PDCD4, and miR-21; it also reduced the ability to generate M2 GAMs. Notably, pacritinib-treated GAMs released fewer miR-21-enriched exosomes. Finally, we demonstrated preclinical support for using pacritinib to overcome TMZ-resistance using a TMZ-resistant LN18-bearing mouse model.

2. Materials and Methods

2.1. Sample Collection and Cell Culture

Tumor sample and stromal GAMs were collected from our Department of Neurosurgery, Taipei Medical University-Shuang Ho Hospital, under strict adherence to Institutional Review Board (IRB) guidelines (approval numbers: IRB: N201801070 and N201602060). Patients were fully informed and a written consent form was signed prior to the operation. The pathological examination was performed by the Department of Pathology and all verified cases met the criteria of GBM. Samples (tumor samples and stromal cells) were isolated and cultured according to previously established protocols [8,9]. Human GBM cell lines U87MG and LN18 were obtained from the American Type Culture Collection (ATCC) and maintained in DMEM supplemented with 2 mM glutamine, 100 U/mL penicillin, 100 µg/mL streptomycin, and 10% FBS. Neurospheres from both cell lines and clinical samples were generated using tumor-sphere-forming medium containing growth factors supplemented with DMEM-F12 1:1 medium, as previously described [10]. For coculture experiments, a previously established protocol was followed with minor modifications [11]. In brief, U87MG and LN18 (2×10^5 cells) were seeded in a transwell insert (0.4 µm pore size) with GAMs (2.5×10^5 cells) seeded in the lower chamber of a six-well system. Cells were cultured in DMEM medium as described above. Cells were maintained for 48 h and harvested for further analyses. In the case of the exosome coculture, GBM cells were cultured in serum-free DMEM in the presence of exosomes for 48 h and harvested.

2.2. Transfection

In order to explore the functional roles of miR-21 in GBM cells, the upregulation or downregulation of miR-21 was achieved using mimic and inhibitor, respectively. MiR-21-5p mimic (HMI0372, Sigma, St. Louis, MO, USA) and inhibitor (HSTUD0371, Sigma, St. Louis, MO, USA) were transfected into GBM cells using Lipofectamine 2000 reagent (Invitrogen, USA) according to the vendor's instructions. The change in the expression of miR-21-5p was then determined by real-time PCR (RT-PCR) 48 h post-transfection in both GBM cell lines. hsa-miR-21-5p primers (MPH02337, Abm, Richmond, BC, Canada) were purchased and used for qPCR experiments.

2.3. Exosome Isolation

GAMs were cultured in serum-free medium for 48 h (with and without pacritinib treatment, 0.5 µM) before exosome isolation. Culture medium was collected and a standard procedure was performed accordingly [12]. In short, we carried out a serial centrifugation procedure ($500 \times g$ for 10 min, $1200 \times g$ for 20 min, and $10,000 \times g$ for 30 min), followed by filtration with a 0.22 µm pore syringe and a spin at $100,000 \times g$ for 60 min. The collected pellet was washed in PBS three times before another ultracentrifugation at $100,000 \times g$ for 60 min. The exosomes were used for further analyses. A small portion of the pellet was processed for transmission electron microscopic examination. In brief, purified exosomes were fixed with 1% glutaraldehyde (1 h, room temperature) and washed, followed by 1% reduced osmium tetroxide fixation (1 h). The sample was washed, stained with 0.3% thiocarbohydrazide, and fixed again in OsO4. Finally, the sample was embedded into Epon. Ultrathin sections were placed on formvar-coated grids. Electron microscopy (EM) analysis was performed as previously described [13]. The flowchart of GBM cell lines either treated with exosomes or mimics or inhibitors is listed in the Supplementary Materials.

2.4. miRNA PCR Array Analysis

Total RNA (200 ng) isolated from exosomes derived from GAMs was transcribed to cDNA using the miScript II RT kit (Qiagen, Valencia, CA, USA) according to the protocol provided by the vendor. The miRNA PCR array (Qiagen, Valencia, CA, USA) was used for profiling according to the instructions provided.

2.5. Real-Time PCR

Total RNAs were extracted, purified, and reverse transcribed using the RNeasy kit (Qiagen, Valencia, CA, USA) and OneStep RT-PCR Kit (Qiagen, Valencia, CA, USA). RT-PCR was performed using an I-Cycler IQ Multicolor RT-PCR Detection System (Bio-Rad) with SsoFast Eva Green Supermix (Bio-Rad). All experimental Ct values were normalized against the Ct value of internal control, GAPDH. Relative abundance was determined by $2-\Delta\Delta Ct$ and expressed as fold changes. Primer sequences are listed in Supplementary Table S1.

2.6. SDS-PAGE and Western Blotting

A standard SDS-PAGE and Western blotting was carried out according to previously established protocols [14]. The primary antibodies used in this study were all purchased from AbCam (Taipei, Taiwan) unless otherwise specified: anti-STAT3 (ab119352, 1:1500); anti-IL-6 (ab6672, 1:500); anti-Sox2 (ab93689, 1:800); anti-Nestin (ab105389, 1:800); anti-CD9 (ab92726, 1:400); anti-CD63 (ab217345, 1:400); anti-CD81 (ab79559. 1:400); anti-actin (ab179467, 1:2000); and anti-tubulin (ab6046, 1:1000).

2.7. In Vivo Xenograft Model

A tumor sample from a GBM patient with TMZ resistance was used to establish the TMZ-resistant mouse model for in vivo evaluation according to previously established protocols [15]. In brief, NOD/SCID mice were anaesthetized (10 mg/kg, ketamine/xylazine and buprenorphine, 0.05 mg/kg, before and after injection). TMZ-resistant LN18 GBM cells (5×10^5 cells) were stereotactically injected into the right striata of the mice. One week postinjection, the mice were randomly divided into vehicle, pacritinib (100 mg/kg, five times/week), TMZ (30 mg/kg, five times/week), or the combination of pacritinib (100 mg/kg) and TMZ (30 mg/kg) groups. Both drugs were administered via oral gavage. Mice were humanely sacrificed by sodium pentobarbital at the end of the experiments. The tumor presence and size were determined in the mice via necropsy and cranial dissection. Tumor samples were harvested for further analysis. The tumor size (average area) was determined from cross sections of the tumor samples. Image J software was used for calculating the tumor size. The animal study protocol was approved by the Animal Care and User Committee at Taipei Medical University (Affidavit of Approval of Animal Use Protocol# Taipei Medical University—LAC-2017-0512).

2.8. Statistical Analysis

The miRNA expression levels from the array experiments were analyzed by SDS software version 2.2.2 (Applied Biosystems, foster city, CA, USA). The delat Ct values were calculated against U6 internal control. Heatmaps of differentially expressed miRNAs were analyzed by R software. Other data were analyzed using Student's *t*-test to determine statistical significance among the different groups. *p*-values (represented by asterisks), where * $p < 0.05$; ** $p < 0.01$; *** $p < 0.001$; **** $p < 0.0001$.

3. Results

3.1. M2 Polarization of GAMs Promotes GBM Tumorigenesis

Initially, we cocultured clinically isolated GAMs with human GBM cell lines U87MG and LN18, which showed increased colony (Figure 1A) and neurosphere (Figure 1B) forming abilities. Consistently, qPCR analysis demonstrated that the presence of GAMs was associated with an increased mRNA level of stemness markers (Figure 1C). The results from the Western blots were consistent where the expression of Sox2, Oct4, Wnt, and Nestin were elevated, while GFAP was decreased in the presence of GAMs (Figure 1D).

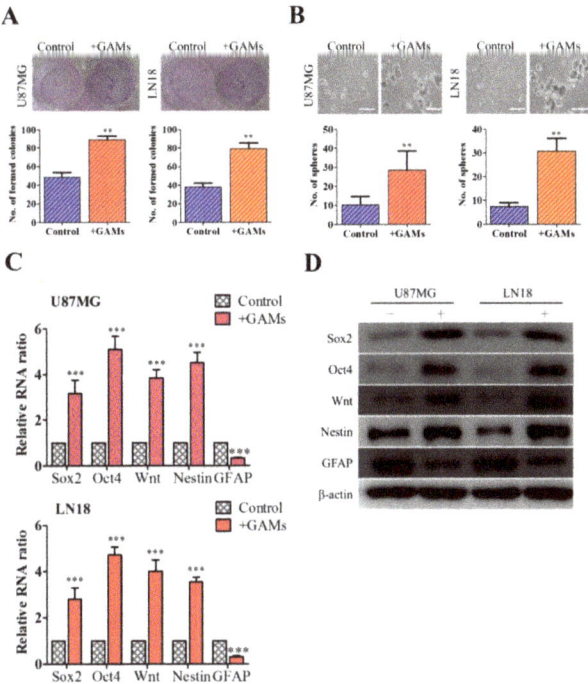

Figure 1. M2 glioblastoma multiforme (GBM)-associated macrophages (GAMs) promote GBM tumorigenesis. GBM cells U87MG and LN18 cocultured with M2 GAMs showed significantly increased colony forming ability (**A**) and tumor sphere generating ability (**B**) as compared to their parental controls. Comparative real-time PCR (**C**) and Western blots (**D**) showed that M2 GAM cocultured GBM cells expressed a significantly higher level of stemness markers, Sox2, Oct4, Wnt, and Nestin while GFAP was reduced. Scale lengths = 100 µm, * $p < 0.05$; ** $p < 0.01$; *** $p < 0.001$.

3.2. Exosome Enriched with miR-21 from GAMs Promotes Tumorigenic Properties

We further investigated the underlying tumorigenesis by isolating and characterizing exosomes secreted into the culture medium by GAMs. First, we used different markers for exosomes—CD9, CD63, and CD81—to verify the identity of the exosomes isolated from the GAMs (Figure 2A). Next, we showed that incubation of GAM-derived exosomes significantly increased TMZ resistance in both U87MG and LN18 cells (Figure 2B). For example, the estimated IC_{50} value for U87MG increased approximately 4-fold after incubation with GAM-derived exosomes, while this was even more significant in the LN18 cells after exosome treatment. This increased TMZ resistance was accompanied by increased colony-forming (Figure 2C) and tumor-sphere-forming (Figure 2D) abilities. We then screened a small cohort of microRNAs in two batches of GAM-derived exosomes and found that miR-21 appeared to be the most abundant microRNA (Figure 2E). As shown in the heatmap, the miR-21 level appeared to be the most enriched in the exosomes collected from two samples of GAMs.

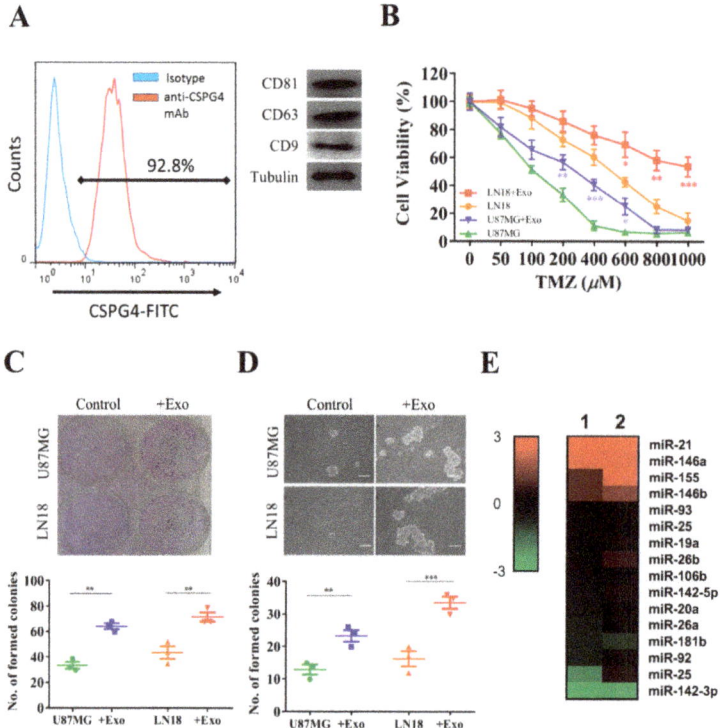

Figure 2. GAM-derived exosomes harbor miR-21, which promote GBM tumorigenesis. (**A**) Representative transmission electronic micrograph of exosomes isolated from clinical GAMs (left); Western blot validation of exosomes isolated from GAM culture medium showed the expression of CD9, CD63, and CD81. (**B**) Increased temozolomide (TMZ) resistance in U87MG and LN18 cells cocultured with exosomes (+exo). Enhanced colony-forming ability (**C**) and tumor-sphere-generating ability (**D**) in the presence GAM-derived exosomes. (**E**) MicroRNA profiling analyses showed that exosomes (two samples) isolated from M2 GAMs contained a high level of miR-21. Scale lengths = 100 μm, * $p < 0.05$; ** $p < 0.01$; *** $p < 0.001$.

3.3. MiR-21 Is Associated with GBM Tumorigenic Properties

Next, we examined the effects of miR-21 on GBM cells by gene silencing and overexpression techniques. First, we demonstrated that miR-21-5p level increased in both U87MG and LN18 cells after being cocultured with GAM-derived exosomes (Figure 3A). We then transfected GBM (postincubation with GAM exosomes) with either mimic or inhibitor molecules of miR-21-5p. We found that the stemness markers Sox2, Oct4, Wnt, STAT3, and Nestin were all significantly increased when mimic miR-21-5p was added to both cells, while the opposite occurred after the miR-21-5p level was inhibited (Figure 3B). The Western blotting results agreed with the real-time PCR results (Figure 3C), where an increased miR-21-5p level led to the increased expression of Sox2, Oct4, STAT3, Akt, Nestin, and Wnt and a decreased level of GFAP. More importantly, tumorigenic properties such as colony formation and tumor sphere formation were also positively correlated with the level of miR-21-5p. For instance, an increased miR-21-5p level by mimic molecules led to an increased number of colonies (Figure 3D) and neurospheres (Figure 3E) generated, and the opposite was true with a decreased level of miR-21-5p with the inhibitor treatment. Furthermore, miR-21-5p mimic transfection made both U87MG and LN18 cells more resistant against TMZ, whereas miR-21-5p inhibitor reversed the resistance (Figure 3F).

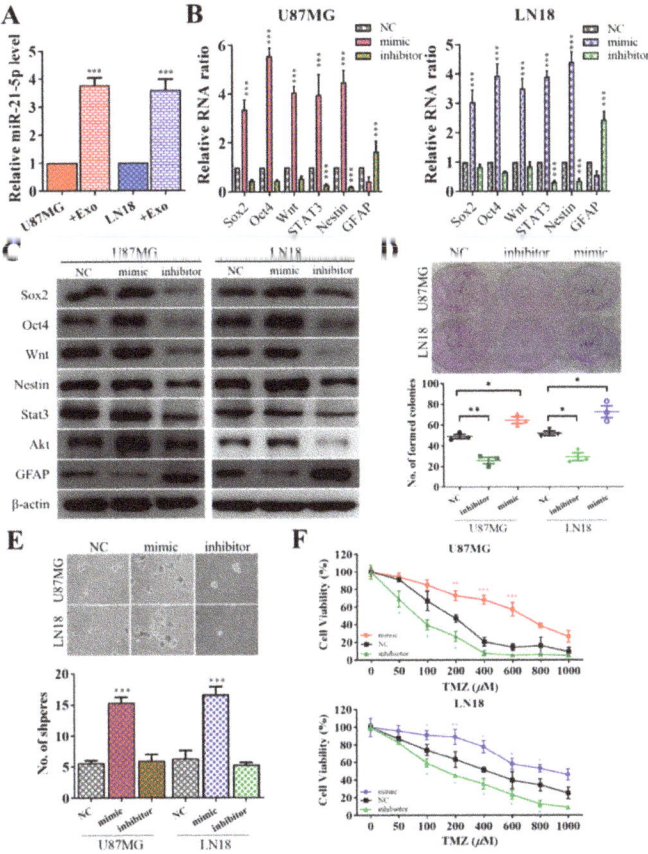

Figure 3. GAM-derived exosomes promoted GBM tumorigenesis via miR-21-5p. (**A**) U87MG and LN18 cells incubated with GAM-derived exosomes showed a significantly increased level of miR-21-5p. GBM tumorigenesis was associated with miR-21-5p. Increased miR-21-5p level (by mimic molecules) in GBM cells showed an increased mRNA level of Sox2, Oct4, Wnt, STAT3, and Nestin or protein level of Sox2, Oct4, STAT3, Akt, Wnt, and Nestin with decreased GFAP, while a decrease in miR-21-5p (inhibitor) led to the opposite phenomenon (**B,C**). Incubation with GAM-derived exosomes increased colony-forming ability (**D**) and tumor-sphere-generating ability (**E**) in both U87MG and LN18 cells. (**F**) U87MG and LN18 cells transfected miR-21-5p mimic molecules (increased miR-21-5p level) resulted in significantly increased TMZ resistance, while there was reduced miR-21-59 and decreased TMZ resistance. Scale lengths = 100 μm, * $p < 0.05$; ** $p < 0.01$; *** $p < 0.001$.

3.4. STAT3 and PDCD4 are Targets of miR-21-5p

Subsequently, we examined the potential target(s) for miR-21-5p using bioinformatics tools and we identified STAT3, a well-known oncogene, and PDCD4, an established tumor suppressor, as the top-ranking candidates from all three algorithms used (PITA, miRmap, and miRanda). A potential site of interaction between miR-21-5p and STAT3 and PDCD4 was identified in the 3′UTR (upper panel, Figure 4A); more importantly, based on TCGA database, a strong negative correlation between the expression level of PDCD4 and miR-21-5p was established within a cohort of GBM patients

(n = 525, lower panel, Figure 4B). We then demonstrated that increased miR-21-5p by mimic molecules in both U87MG and LN18 cells supported the negative correlation between the expression of miR-21-5p and PDCD4. Conversely, a decreased level of miR-21-5p by inhibitor molecules restored the expression of PDCD4 (Figure 4C). We then cocultured miR-21-5p-silenced GBM cells with GAMs and observed a significantly reduced M2 signature (CD68+/CD206+) (Figure 4D). More importantly, the M2 cytokines VEGF, TGF-β1, and IL-6 released by GAMs cocultured with miR-21-5p-silenced U87MG cells were significantly reduced and restored partially after cocultured miR-21-5p-silenced U87MG were transfected with mimic of miR-21-5p (Figure 4E).

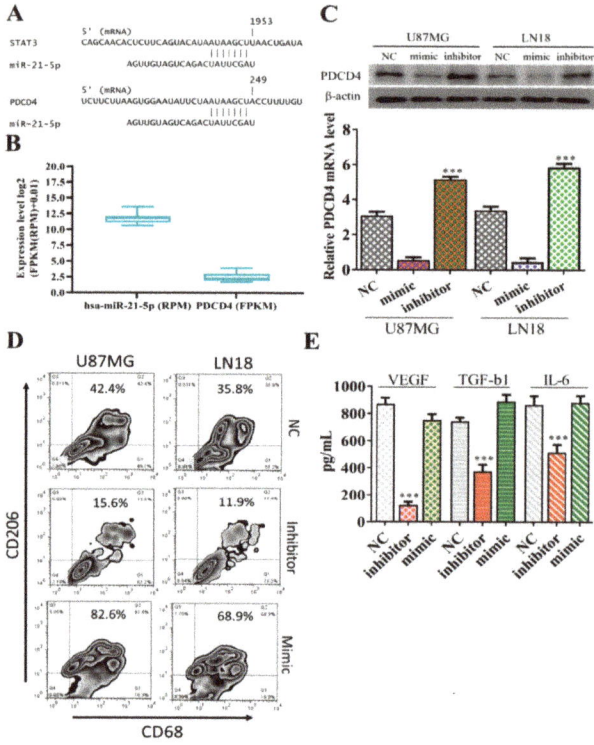

Figure 4. MiR-21-5p targets STAT3 and PDCD4. (**A**) The bioinformatics tool shows miR-21-5p binding to the 3′UTR of STAT3 and PDCD4 (upper panel). (**B**) A negative correlation between the expression of miR-21-5p and PDCD4 in the GBM database (n = 525, TCGA). (**C**) An increased miR-21-5p level (by mimic molecule, lane M) led to significantly reduced PDCD4 expression in both U87MG and LN18 cells; the reverse was true with the inhibitor of miR-21-5p. (**D**) Flow cytometry analysis showed a significantly reduced CD206$^+$/CD68$^+$ population in GAMs cocultured with miR-21-5p-silenced U87MG and LN18 cells; the reverse was observed in miR-21-5p mimic transfected coculture experiments. (**E**) The inhibitor of miR-21-5p resulted in the reduction of VEGF, TGF- β1, and IL-6 secreted by the U87MG cells into the culture medium. *** $p < 0.001$.

3.5. Pacritinib Suppresses GBM Tumorigenesis and M2 Polarization of GAMs

Elevated STAT3 signaling has been attributed to the malignancy of GBM and the generation of glioma stem cells [16]. In addition, increased STAT3 signaling is associated with the increased miR-21 level in the promotion of tumorigenesis [17,18]. Based on these premises, we examined a clinical STAT3 inhibitor, pacritinib, for its potential GBM inhibitory effects. We found that pacritinib treatment significantly suppressed the cell viability of both U87MG and LN18 cells at low IC$_{50}$ values

(0.5 and 1.7 µM, respectively) (Figure 5A). Subsequently, we showed that pacritinib-treated U87MG and LN18 cells contained a significantly lower ability to generate M2-polarized GAMs (Figure 5B), as reflected by the reduced CD206 (M2 marker) and increased TNF-α (M1 marker). In addition, the addition of pacritinib prominently suppressed colony formation (Figure 5C) and tumor sphere generation (Figure 5D). Furthermore, pacritinib treatment led to a decreased expression of Sox2, PDCD4, and STAT3; more importantly, the level of miR-21-5p in both GBM cell lines was suppressed as well (Figure 5E). Notably, pacritinib treatment led to significantly reduced exosome release and a corresponding level of miR-21-5p from GAMs (Figure 5F).

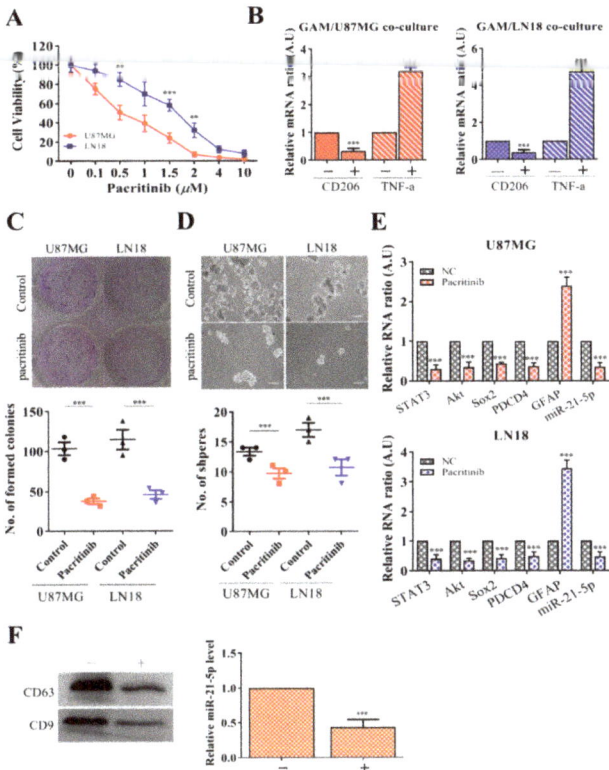

Figure 5. Pacritinib treatment suppresses GBM tumorigenesis and glioma stem cell (GSC) properties. (**A**) Pacritinib treatment significantly suppressed both U87MG and LN18 cells (approximate IC$_{50}$ values 0.5 and 1.5 µM, respectively). (**B**) Pacritinib treatment significantly reduced GBM cells' ability to induce M2 GAMs. CD206 mRNA in GAMs was significantly reduced, while TNF-α was increased. Pacritinib treatment significantly reduced colony formation (**C**) and tumor sphere generation (**D**) in both U87MG and LN18 cells. (**E**) Pacritinib treatment led to a significantly reduced mRNA level of STAT3, Akt, Sox2, PDCD4, and miR-21-5p and increased GFAP in both U87MG and LN18 cells. (**F**) GAMs treated with pacritinib resulted in the decreased release of exosomes. Western blot of exosomes collected from GAMs showed a significantly lower abundance of exosomes (CD63 and CD9, markers of exosomes). The exosomes collected showed a significantly lower miR-21-5p level. Scale lengths = 100 µm, * $p < 0.05$; ** $p < 0.01$; *** $p < 0.001$.

3.6. In Vivo Evaluation of Pacritinib

Finally, we evaluated the potential of using pacritinib as a treatment for GBM using a preclinical mouse model bearing TMZ-resistant LN18 cells (cocultured with exosomes isolated from GAMs).

Representative brain slices showed that a single treatment of pacritinib suppressed the tumorigenesis of TMZ-resistant LN18 cells compared to TMZ single treatment and vehicle control (Figure 6A). Notably, there was no significant difference in tumor size between vehicle control and TMZ single treatment groups (Figure 6B), while the combination of pacritinib and TMZ appeared to produce the most significant inhibitory effect on tumor progression (right panel, Figure 6B). In support, tumor samples harvested from the combination of pacritinib and TMZ showed the lowest level of STAT3, Sox2, PDCD4, and miR-21-5p and an increased level of GFAP (Figure 6C). Microglial cells isolated from the single pacritinib treatment and the combination of pacritinib and TMZ groups also demonstrated a significantly reduced CD206 mRNA level and an increased TNF-α level (Figure 6D). The overall median survival was significantly increased in each treatment group compared with vehicle control (Figure 6E). Median survival was 19 days for vehicle control, 24 days for TMZ ($p = 0.024$, compared with control), 26.5 days for pacritinib ($p = 0.0098$, compared with control), and 32.5 day for combination of pacritinib and TMZ ($p = 0.0006$, compared with control, $p = 0.0092$, compared with TMZ, $p = 0.0219$, compared with pacritinib) (Figure 6F).

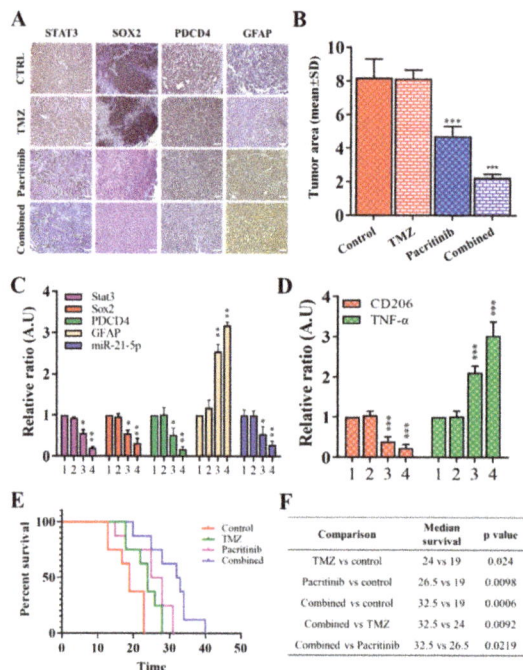

Figure 6. In vivo evaluation of pacritinib for treating GBM and reducing M2 GAMs in TMZ-resistant LN18 bearing mice. (**A**) Immunohistochemical staining in TMZ-resistant LN18-bearing mice showed that treatment in the pacritinib group and pacritinib/TMZ combination group suppressed tumorigenesis. (**B**) The tumor size showed that the significantly reduced tumor size in the pacritinib group and the combination of pacritinib and TMZ group led to the most significantly reduced tumor size. NS, statistically nonsignificant. (**C**) Comparative real-time PCR analyses showed the reduced mRNA level of STAT3, Sox2, PDCD4, and miR-21-5p and the increased GFAP expression in the pacritinib group and pacritinib/TMZ combination group (lane 1, control; lane 2, TMZ alone; lane 3, pacritinib alone; lane 4, pacritinib/TMZ combination). (**D**) M2 GAMs from tumor samples showed a significantly reduced CD206 (M2 marker) mRNA level (lane 3, pacritinib alone; lane 4, pacritinib/TMZ combination) and an increase in TNF-α (lanes 3 and 4). (**E**) Kaplan–Meier survival curve and (**F**) statistical comparisons showed increased median overall survival in TMZ, pacritinib, and pacritinib/TMZ combination groups. Scale lengths = 50 µm, * $p < 0.05$; ** $p < 0.01$; *** $p < 0.001$.

4. Discussion

Despite advances in therapeutics development over the past decade, GBM remains challenging to treat due to its heterogeneity and malignant nature. The tumor microenvironment plays a crucial role in promoting GBM tumorigenesis. GAMs have been shown to be one of the key players in the GBM microenvironment. We first demonstrated that clinical samples of GAMs promoted GBM tumorigenesis. For instance, U87MG and LN18 GBM cells cocultured with clinical M2 GAMs showed increased colony-forming and tumor-sphere-generating abilities in association with increased stemness markers Sox2, STAT3, Wnt, and Nestin in the GBM cells. Accumulating evidence has supported the observations where GAMs induced epithelial–mesenchymal transition (EMT) in GBM cells and subsequently generated properties of GSCs [19]. In addition, our observations were in agreement with previous studies, where interactions between GBM and GAMs increased CD133+ GSCs and malignant phenotypes [20,21]. GAM-mediated GBM-promoting effects were through different communicating molecules such as M2 cytokines (IL-6, VEGF, and TGF-β1) [2]. Here, we showed that the presence of GAMs promoted GBM tumorigenesis and stemness not only via the cytokines but also through the aid of exosomes. More specifically, we found that GBM cells incubated with exosomes derived from GAMs exhibited enhanced ability in colony and tumor sphere formation; more importantly, exosome-incubated GBM cells became more resistant against TMZ. Emerging evidence indicates the functional roles of exosomes in GBM tumorigenesis. A recent study showed that exosomes secreted from GBM cells promoted the oncogenic transformation of astrocytes in the tumor microenvironment [22]. This observation complements the results of our study, which demonstrated intimate communication between the tumor microenvironment and tumor cells via the exchange of exosomes.

We performed an array analysis on the exosomes secreted by GAMs and found that the most abundant microRNA species was miR-21. Notably, a recent review points out that miR-21 plays a pivotal role in GBM pathogenesis, where miR-21 functions through the modulation of the insulin-like-growth-factor-associated signaling pathway, RECK, and TIMP3 to promote GBM tumorigenesis [23]. Our results provided an added feature of miR-21 in GBM tumorigenesis, where miR-21 was enriched in the exosomes secreted by GAMs. It is very plausible that GAM-derived miR-21-enriched exosomes were incorporated into GBM cells and executed their tumor-promoting functions. It has been well demonstrated that the transfer and uptake of exosomes between donor and recipient cells represents one of the major routes for intercellular communications in many diseases, including cancer [24]. We provided support that increased miR-21-5p in GBM cells by miR-21-5p mimic molecules resulted in similar tumorigenic and stemness properties in GBM cells cocultured with GAM-derived exosomes; the reduction of miR-21-5p significantly reduced the tumorigenic properties in both GBM cell lines. Furthermore, GBM cells transfected with miR-21-5p inhibitor showed a significantly reduced ability to generate M2 GAMs, based on our coculture experiments; this was attributed to the decreased secretion of M2 cytokines such as IL-6 and VEGF by miR-21-5p-silenced GBM cells and an increased secretion of TNF-α, an M1 marker. More importantly, we provided evidence that miR-21-5p targets PDCD4, a tumor suppressor in both GBM cell lines. PDCD4 has been shown to be frequently suppressed in GBM cells and is associated with poor prognosis [25,26]. In agreement with our results, a previous study also demonstrated that PDCD4 was targeted by miR-21 in GBM [27].

According to our experimental results, miR-416a ranks as the second-most abundant microRNA species in the GAM-secreted exosomes. It has been shown that miR-416a plays a key role in the progression of malignant melanoma via the activation of notch signaling [28]. The activation of notch signaling has also been shown to be responsible for the generation of GSCs [29,30]. The fact that miR-21 and miR-416a, two powerful oncogenic microRNA molecules, were enriched in the GAM exosomes further supports our notion that GAMs play a key contributing role in GBM malignancy and should be targeted in treatment design. Currently, the role of exosomal miR-416a in GBM tumorigenesis is under intense investigation in our laboratory.

Since targeting microRNA for therapeutic purposes still remains challenging, miR-21-5p represents a potential therapeutic target. Thus, we evaluated the feasibility of using a small-molecule agent which may indirectly increase the miR-21 level to convey therapeutic functions in GBM. STAT3 signaling has been shown to be important in GBM tumorigenesis as well as linked to the expression of miR-21 [17,31,32]. Based on these premises, we evaluated pacritinib, a recent FDA-approved inhibitor of STAT3/JAK2 signaling for treating myelofibrosis [33,34]. We found pacritinib treatment suppressed cell viability and colony/tumor sphere formation in association with decreased expression of STAT3, Sox2, PDCD4, and miR-21-5p and increased GFAP expression. Equally important, GAMs cocultured with pacritinib-treated U87MG and LN18 GBM cells showed a significantly reduced M2 marker (CD206) and increased M1 marker (TNF-α), strongly suggesting pacritinib not only suppressed GBM tumorigenesis but also affected GAM polarization. These tumor inhibitory and tumor microenvironment normalizing effects of pacritinib could be attributed to the suppression of STAT3/JAK2 signaling. Our observations were supported by a recent report that the inhibition of the JAK/STAT3 pathway resulted in disrupted intercellular communications between microglia and GBM cells [35] and pronounced anti-GBM effects [36,37]. In addition, we found that pacritinib treatment was able to suppress the number of miR-21-enriched exosomes secreted by GAMs.

Finally, we provided support for combining pacritinib with TMZ using a TMZ-resistant GBM mouse model. A single treatment of pacritinib was sufficient to suppress GBM growth, while the combination of pacritinib and TMZ exerted the most significant inhibitory effect. Several studies have demonstrated the benefit of using a STAT3 inhibitor to overcome TMZ resistance [38,39]. Notably, one report showed that STAT3 inhibitor treatment promoted the infiltration of tumoricidal lymphocytes [40]. Another study also lends support to our results, where the sequential combination of STAT3 inhibition and TMZ led to the induction of GBM apoptosis with an increased level of miR-21 [41]. This is consistent with another previous study that combined treatment with pacritinib and TMZ to dramatically reduce the activity of the JAK2/STAT3 pathway. This highlights the potential for pacritinib to be a useful adjuvant therapy with the standard-of-care TMZ. Additionally, pacritinib could be used as a salvage therapy for patients with a TMZ-resistant recurrent disease, as STAT3 inhibition sensitizes TMZ-resistant, patient-derived brain-tumor-initiating cell (BTIC) cultures [42].

5. Conclusions

In conclusion, as shown in the scheme in Figure 7, we have provided translational evidence that miR-21-enriched GAM-derived exosomes contribute to GBM malignancy via increasing stemness. The feasibility of using pacritinib to modulate STAT3/miR-21/PDCD4 signaling was demonstrated using both in vitro and in vivo GBM models. Further investigation is warranted for conducting potential clinical trials for GBM patients experiencing TMZ resistance.

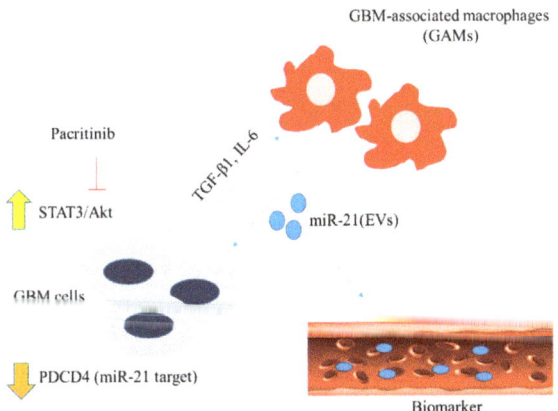

Figure 7. GAMs in the tumor microenvironment promote the survival of GBM cells via miR-21-enriched extracellular microvesicles (EVs). Mir-21 targets and suppresses the expression of tumor suppressor PDCD4 in GBM cells, leading to the elevated STAT3/Akt signaling. In turn, GBM cells secrete inflammatory cytokines TGF-β1 and IL-6 and promote M2 polarization. Pacritinib (STAT3 inhibitor) treatment suppresses GBM tumorigenesis by inhibiting STAT3 signaling and reducing M2 polarization of GAMs.

6. Ethics Approval and Consent to Participate

Clinical samples were collected from Taipei Medical University (Taipei, Taiwan). All enrolled patients gave written informed consent for their tissues to be used for scientific research. The study was approved by the IRB of the Taipei Medical University (IRB: N201801070 and N201602060), consistent with the recommendations of the Declaration of Helsinki for biomedical research (Taipei Medical University (Taipei, Taiwan) and following standard institutional protocol for human research. Moreover, the animal study protocol was approved by the Animal Care and User Committee at Taipei Medical University (Taipei, Taiwan) (Affidavit of Approval of Animal Use Protocol# Taipei Medical University—LAC-2017-0512).

Supplementary Materials: The following are available online at http://www.mdpi.com/2077-0383/8/7/959/s1, Supplementary Materials: Figure S1: Full-size blots of Figure 1D, Figure S2: Full-size blots of Figure 2A, Figure S3: Full-size blots of Figure 3C, Figure S4: Full-size blots of Figure 4C, Figure S5: Full-size blots of Figure 5F, Figure S6: Flowchart of GBM cell lines and GAMs from clinical human GBM specimen isolation, Figure S7: Flowchart of exosome isolation, Figure S8: Flowchart of GBM cell lines either treated with exosomes or mimics or inhibitors, Table S1. Primer sequences used in this study, Table S2. Western blot antibody sheet.

Author Contributions: Conceived and designed the study: H.-Y.C. and Y.-K.S. Performed the experiments: H.-W.L. and C.-H.C. Analyzed the data: S.-C.C. and D.-Y.C. Bioinformatics: S.-Z.L. Wrote the manuscript: H.-Y.C. and Y.-K.S. Provided reagents, materials, experimental infrastructure, and administrative oversight: Y.-S.C. and C.-M.L. All authors read and approved the final version of the manuscript.

Funding: This work was supported by the National Science Council of Taiwan grant to Chien-Min Lin (MOST 107-2314-B-038 –056 -MY3) and grants to Yu-Kai Su (MOST 107-2314-B-038-022). This study was also supported by grants from Taipei Medical University, Taiwan (106-FRP-03) to Chien-Min Lin.

Acknowledgments: The authors thank the laboratory assistant Mr. Iat-Hang Fong (Department of Medical Research and Education, Taipei Medical University-Shuang Ho Hospital) for his technical assistance.

Conflicts of Interest: The authors declare that they have no potential financial competing interests from which they may in any way gain or lose financially from the publication of this manuscript presently or in the future. Additionally, no nonfinancial competing interests are involved in the manuscript.

Abbreviations

M2 GAMs	M2 polarization of glioblastoma associated macrophages
NC	negative controls
GBM	glioblastoma multiforme
TMZ	temozolomide
GSCs	glioma stem cells
lncRNAs	long noncoding RNAs
IRB	Institutional Review Board
TME	tumor microenvironment

References

1. Khosla, D. Concurrent therapy to enhance radiotherapeutic outcomes in glioblastoma. *Ann. Transl. Med.* **2016**, *4*, 5.
2. Hambardzumyan, D.; Gutmann, D.H.; Kettenmann, H. The role of microglia and macrophages in glioma maintenance and progression. *Nat. Neurosci.* **2016**, *19*, 20–27. [CrossRef] [PubMed]
3. Bowman, R.L.; A Joyce, J. Therapeutic targeting of tumor-associated macrophages and microglia in glioblastoma. *Immunother.* **2014**, *6*, 663–666. [CrossRef] [PubMed]
4. Skog, J.; Würdinger, T.; Van Rijn, S.; Meijer, D.H.; Gainche, L.; Curry, W.T.; Carter, B.S.; Krichevsky, A.M.; Breakefield, X.O.; Sena-Esteves, M.; et al. Glioblastoma microvesicles transport RNA and proteins that promote tumour growth and provide diagnostic biomarkers. *Nat. Cell Biol.* **2008**, *10*, 1470–1476. [CrossRef] [PubMed]
5. Graner, M.W.; Cumming, R.I.; Bigner, D.D. The Heat Shock Response and Chaperones/Heat Shock Proteins in Brain Tumors: Surface Expression, Release, and Possible Immune Consequences. *J. Neurosci.* **2007**, *27*, 11214–11227. [CrossRef] [PubMed]
6. Murgoci, A.-N.; Cízková, D.; Majerova, P.; Petrovová, E.; Medvecký, L'.; Fournier, I.; Salzet, M. Brain-Cortex Microglia-Derived Exosomes: Nanoparticles for Glioma Therapy. *ChemPhysChem* **2018**, *19*, 1205–1214. [CrossRef]
7. Caccese, M.; Indraccolo, S.; Zagonel, V.; Lombardi, G.; Mario, C.; Giuseppe, L.; Stefano, I.; Vittorina, Z. PD-1/PD-L1 immune-checkpoint inhibitors in glioblastoma: A concise review. *Crit. Rev. Oncol.* **2019**, *135*, 128–134. [CrossRef]
8. Stechishin, O.D.; Luchman, H.A.; Ruan, Y.; Blough, M.D.; Nguyen, S.A.; Kelly, J.J.; Cairncross, J.G.; Weiss, S. On-target JAK2/STAT3 inhibition slows disease progression in orthotopic xenografts of human glioblastoma brain tumor stem cells. *Neuro-Oncology* **2013**, *15*, 198–207. [CrossRef]
9. Kelly, J.J.P.; Stechishin, O.; Chojnacki, A.; Lun, X.; Sun, B.; Senger, D.L.; Forsyth, P.; Auer, R.N.; Dunn, J.F.; Cairncross, J.G.; et al. Proliferation of Human Glioblastoma Stem Cells Occurs Independently of Exogenous Mitogens. *Stem Cells* **2009**, *27*, 1722–1733. [CrossRef]
10. Ortensi, B.; Osti, D.; Pellegatta, S.; Pisati, F.; Brescia, P.; Fornasari, L.; Levi, D.; Gaetani, P.; Colombo, P.; Ferri, A.; et al. Rai is a New Regulator of Neural Progenitor Migration and Glioblastoma Invasion. *Stem Cells* **2012**, *30*, 817–832. [CrossRef]
11. Gagliano; Costa, F.; Cossetti, C.; Pettinari, L.; Bassi, R.; Chiriva-Internati, M.; Cobos, E.; Gioia, M.; Pluchino, S. Glioma-astrocyte interaction modifies the astrocyte phenotype in a co-culture experimental model. *Oncol. Rep.* **2009**, *22*, 1349–1356. [CrossRef]
12. Thery, C.; Amigorena, S.; Raposo, G.; Clayton, A. Isolation and characterization of exosomes from cell culture supernatants and biological fluids. *Curr. Protoc. Cell Biol.* **2006**, *3*. [CrossRef] [PubMed]
13. Beznoussenko, G.V.; Dolgikh, V.V.; Seliverstova, E.V.; Semenov, P.B.; Tokarev, Y.S.; Trucco, A.; Micaroni, M.; Di Giandomenico, D.; Auinger, P.; Senderskiy, I.V.; et al. Analogs of the Golgi complex in microsporidia: structure and avesicular mechanisms of function. *J. Cell Sci.* **2007**, *120*, 1288–1298. [CrossRef] [PubMed]
14. Mahmood, T.; Yang, P.-C. Western Blot: Technique, Theory, and Trouble Shooting. *North Am. J. Med Sci.* **2012**, *4*, 429–434.
15. Carlson, B.L.; Pokorny, J.L.; Schroeder, M.A.; Sarkaria, J.N. Establishment, Maintenance and in vitro and in vivo Applications of Primary Human Glioblastoma Multiforme (GBM) Xenograft Models for Translational Biology Studies and Drug Discovery. *Curr. Protocols Pharmacol.* **2011**, *52*, 1–14.

16. Ganguly, D.; Fan, M.; Yang, C.H.; Zbytek, B.; Finkelstein, D.; Roussel, M.F.; Pfeffer, L.M. The critical role that STAT3 plays in glioma-initiating cells: STAT3 addiction in glioma. *Oncotarget* **2018**, *9*, 22095–22112. [CrossRef]
17. Chen, N.; Feng, L.; Qu, H.; Lu, K.; Li, P.; Lv, X.; Wang, X. Overexpression of IL-9 induced by STAT3 phosphorylation is mediated by miR-155 and miR-21 in chronic lymphocytic leukemia. *Oncology reports* **2018**, *39*, 3064–3072. [CrossRef]
18. Zhou, J.; Li, X.; Wu, X.; Zhang, T.; Zhu, Q.; Wang, X.; Wang, H.; Wang, K.; Lin, Y.; Wang, X. Exosomes Released from Tumor-Associated Macrophages Transfer miRNAs That Induce a Treg/Th17 Cell Imbalance in Epithelial Ovarian Cancer. *Cancer Immunol. Res.* **2018**, *6*, 1578–1592. [CrossRef]
19. Harris, M.A.; Yang, H.; Low, B.E.; Mukherje, J.; Guha, A.; Bronson, R.T.; Shultz, L.D.; Israel, M.A.; Yun, K. Cancer stem cells are enriched in the side-population cells in a mouse model of glioma. *Cancer Res.* **2008**, *68*, 10051–10059. [CrossRef]
20. Yao, Y.; Ye, H.; Qi, Z.; Mo, L.; Yue, Q.; Baral, A.; Hoon, D.S.; Vera, J.C.; Heiss, J.D.; Chen, C.C.; et al. B7-H4(B7x)-mediated cross-talk between glioma initiating cells and macrophages via the IL-6/JAK/STAT3 pathway lead to poor prognosis in glioma patients. *Clin. Cancer Res.* **2016**, *22*, 2778–2790. [CrossRef]
21. Zhou, W.; Ke, S.Q.; Huang, Z.; Flavahan, W.; Fang, X.; Paul, J.; Wu, L.; Sloan, A.E.; McLendon, R.E.; Li, X.; et al. Periostin secreted by glioblastoma stem cells recruits M2 tumour-associated macrophages and promotes malignant growth. *Nat. Cell Biol.* **2015**, *17*, 170–182. [CrossRef] [PubMed]
22. Oushy, S.; Hellwinkel, J.E.; Wang, M.; Nguyen, G.J.; Gunaydin, D.; Harland, T.A.; Anchordoquy, T.J.; Graner, M.W. Glioblastoma multiforme-derived extracellular vesicles drive normal astrocytes towards a tumour-enhancing phenotype. Philosophical transactions of the Royal Society of London. *Biologic. Sci.* **2018**, *373*. [CrossRef]
23. Masoudi, M.S.; Mehrabian, E.; Mirzaei, H. MiR-21: A key player in glioblastoma pathogenesis. *J. Cell. Biochem.* **2018**, *119*, 1285–1290. [CrossRef] [PubMed]
24. Ruivo, C.F.; Adem, B.; Silva, M.; Melo, S.A. The Biology of Cancer Exosomes: Insights and New Perspectives. *Cancer Res.* **2017**, *77*, 6480–6488. [CrossRef] [PubMed]
25. Gao, F.; Wang, X.; Zhu, F.; Wang, Q.; Zhang, X.; Guo, C.; Zhou, C.; Ma, C.; Sun, W.; Zhang, Y.; et al. PDCD4 gene silencing in gliomas is associated with 5′CpG island methylation and unfavourable prognosis. *J. Cell. Mol. Med.* **2009**, *13*, 4257–4267. [CrossRef] [PubMed]
26. Gao, F.; Zhang, P.; Zhou, C.; Li, J.; Wang, Q.; Zhu, F.; Ma, C.; Sun, W.; Zhang, L. Frequent loss of PDCD4 expression in human glioma: Possible role in the tumorigenesis of glioma. *Oncol. Rep.* **2007**, *17*, 123–128. [CrossRef] [PubMed]
27. Wang, G.; Wang, J.J.; Tang, H.M.; To, S.S.T. Targeting strategies on miRNA-21 and PDCD4 for glioblastoma. *Arch. Biochem. Biophys.* **2015**, *580*, 64–74. [CrossRef]
28. Forloni, M.; Dogra, S.K.; Dong, Y.; Conte, D.; Ou, J.; Zhu, L.J.; Deng, A.; Mahalingam, M.; Green, M.R.; Wajapeyee, N. miR-146a promotes the initiation and progression of melanoma by activating Notch signaling. *eLife* **2014**, *3*, e01460. [CrossRef]
29. Popescu, I.-D.; Codrici, E.; Enciu, A.-M.; Mihai, S.; Tanase, C. Glioma Stem Cells and Their Microenvironments: Providers of Challenging Therapeutic Targets. *Stem Cells Int.* **2016**, *2016*, 5728438.
30. Ma, Y.; Cheng, Z.; Liu, J.; Torre-Healy, L.; Lathia, J.D.; Nakano, I.; Guo, Y.; Thompson, R.C.; Freeman, M.L.; Wang, J. Inhibition of Farnesyltransferase Potentiates NOTCH-Targeted Therapy against Glioblastoma Stem Cells. *Stem Cell Rep.* **2017**, *9*, 1948–1960. [CrossRef]
31. Gutsaeva, D.R.; Thounaojam, M.; Rajpurohit, S.; Powell, F.L.; Martin, P.M.; Goei, S.; Duncan, M.; Bartoli, M. STAT3-mediated activation of miR-21 is involved in down-regulation of TIMP3 and neovascularization in the ischemic retina. *Oncotarget* **2017**, *8*, 103568–103580. [CrossRef] [PubMed]
32. Ning, S.-L.; Zhu, H.; Shao, J.; Liu, Y.-C.; Lan, J.; Miao, J. MiR-21 inhibitor improves locomotor function recovery by inhibiting IL-6R/JAK-STAT pathway-mediated inflammation after spinal cord injury in model of rat. *Eur. Rev. Med Pharmacol. Sci.* **2019**, *23*, 433–440.
33. Betts, B.C.; Bastian, D.; Iamsawat, S.; Nguyen, H.; Heinrichs, J.L.; Wu, Y.; Daenthanasanmak, A.; Veerapathran, A.; O'Mahony, A.; Walton, K.; et al. Targeting JAK2 reduces GVHD and xenograft rejection through regulation of T cell differentiation. *Proc. Natl. Acad. Sci. USA* **2018**, *115*, 1582–1587. [CrossRef] [PubMed]

34. Mascarenhas, J.; Hoffman, R.; Talpaz, M.; Gerds, A.T.; Stein, B.; Gupta, V.; Szoke, A.; Drummond, M.; Pristupa, A.; Granston, T.; et al. Pacritinib vs Best Available Therapy, Including Ruxolitinib, in Patients With Myelofibrosis: A Randomized Clinical Trial. *JAMA Oncol.* **2018**, *4*, 652–659. [CrossRef] [PubMed]
35. Couto, M.; Coelho-Santos, V.; Santos, L.; Fontes-Ribeiro, C.; Silva, A.P.; Gomes, C.M.F. The Interplay between Glioblastoma and Microglia Cells Leads to Endothelial Cell Monolayer Dysfunction via the Interleukin-6-Induced JAK2/STAT3 Pathway. Available online: https://onlinelibrary.wiley.com/doi/abs/10.1002/jcp.28575 (accessed on 26 May 2019).
36. Linder, B.; Weirauch, U.; Ewe, A.; Uhmann, A.; Seifert, V.; Mittelbronn, M.; Harter, P.N.; Aigner, A.; Kögel, D. Therapeutic Targeting of Stat3 Using Lipopolyplex Nanoparticle-Formulated siRNA in a Syngeneic Orthotopic Mouse Glioma Model. *Cancers* **2019**, *11*, 333. [CrossRef] [PubMed]
37. Liu, T.; Li, A.; Xu, Y.; Xin, Y. Momelotinib sensitizes glioblastoma cells to temozolomide by enhancement of autophagy via JAK2/STAT3 inhibition. *Oncol. Rep.* **2019**, *41*, 1883–1892. [CrossRef] [PubMed]
38. Ashizawa, T.; Akiyama, Y.; Miyata, H.; Iizuka, A.; Komiyama, M.; Kume, A.; Omiya, M.; Sugino, T.; Asai, A.; Hayashi, N.; et al. Effect of the STAT3 inhibitor STX-0119 on the proliferation of a temozolomide-resistant glioblastoma cell line. *Int. J. Oncol.* **2014**, *45*, 411–418. [CrossRef]
39. Miyata, H.; Ashizawa, T.; Iizuka, A.; Kondou, R.; Nonomura, C.; Sugino, T.; Urakami, K.; Asai, A.; Hayashi, N.; Mitsuya, K.; et al. Combination of a STAT3 Inhibitor and an mTOR Inhibitor Against a Temozolomide-resistant Glioblastoma Cell Line. *Cancer Genom. Proteom.* **2017**, *14*, 83–91. [CrossRef]
40. Akiyama, Y.; Nonomura, C.; Ashizawa, T.; Iizuka, A.; Kondou, R.; Miyata, H.; Sugino, T.; Mitsuya, K.; Hayashi, N.; Nakasu, Y.; et al. The anti-tumor activity of the STAT3 inhibitor STX-0119 occurs via promotion of tumor-infiltrating lymphocyte accumulation in temozolomide-resistant glioblastoma cell line. *Immunol. Lett.* **2017**, *190*, 20–25. [CrossRef]
41. Qian, X.; Long, L.; Pu, P.; Ren, Y.; Shi, Z.; Sheng, J.; Yuan, X.; Kang, C. Sequence-Dependent Synergistic Inhibition of Human Glioma Cell Lines by Combined Temozolomide and miR-21 Inhibitor Gene Therapy. *Mol. Pharm.* **2012**, *9*, 2636–2645. [CrossRef]
42. Jensen, K.V.; Cseh, O.; Aman, A.; Weiss, S.; Luchman, H.A. The JAK2/STAT3 inhibitor pacritinib effectively inhibits patient-derived GBM brain tumor initiating cells in vitro and when used in combination with temozolomide increases survival in an orthotopic xenograft model. *PLos ONE* **2017**, *12*, e0189670. [CrossRef] [PubMed]

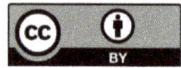

© 2019 by the authors. Licensee MDPI, Basel, Switzerland. This article is an open access article distributed under the terms and conditions of the Creative Commons Attribution (CC BY) license (http://creativecommons.org/licenses/by/4.0/).

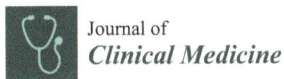

Article

Analysis of Tumor Angiogenesis and Immune Microenvironment in Non-Functional Pituitary Endocrine Tumors

Mizuto Sato, Ryota Tamura, Haruka Tamura, Taro Mase, Kenzo Kosugi, Yukina Morimoto, Kazunari Yoshida and Masahiro Toda *

Department of Neurosurgery, Keio University School of Medicine, 35 Shinanomachi, Shinjuku-ku, Tokyo 160 8582, Japan; mizuto.sato@gmail.com (M.S.); multobello-r-010@hotmail.co.jp (R.T.); rovin124th@gmail.com (H.T.); mstr.komed05241996@gmail.com (T.M.); kensan03977@yahoo.co.jp (K.K.); yukinaxnashiko@yahoo.co.jp (Y.M.); kazrmky@keio.jp (K.Y.)
* Correspondence: todam@keio.jp; Tel.: +81-3-3353-1211

Received: 15 April 2019; Accepted: 14 May 2019; Published: 16 May 2019

Abstract: Cavernous sinus (CS) invasion is an aggressive behavior exhibited by pituitary neuroendocrine tumors (PitNETs). The cause of CS invasion in PitNETs has not been fully elucidated. The tumor immune microenvironment, known to promote aggressive behavior in various types of tumors, has not been examined for PitNETs. Vascular endothelial growth factor (VEGF)/VEGF receptor (VEGFR) signaling is strongly associated with the tumor immune microenvironment. In the present study, these molecular and histopathological characteristics were examined in invasive non-functional PitNETs (NF-PitNETs). Twenty-seven patients with newly diagnosed NF-PitNETs (with CS invasion: 17, without CS invasion: 10) were analyzed by immunohistochemistry for VEGF-A/VEGFR1 and 2, hypoxia-inducible Factor (HIF), tumor-infiltrating lymphocytes, immunosuppressive cells including regulatory T cells (Tregs) and tumor-associated macrophages (TAMs), and immune checkpoint molecules. Previously validated tumor proliferation markers including mitotic count, Ki-67 index, and p53 were also analyzed for their expressions in NF-PitNETs. VEGF-A and VEGFR1 were expressed on not only vascular endothelial cells, but also on tumor cells. The expressions of VEGF-A and VEGFR1 were significantly higher in NF-PitNETs with CS invasion. The number of TAMs and the expression of PD-L1 were also significantly higher in NF-PitNETs with CS invasion than in NF-PitNETs without CS invasion. The high expression of VEGF-A and VEGFR1 and associated immunosuppressive microenvironment were observed in NF-PitNETs with CS invasion, suggesting that a novel targeted therapy can be applied.

Keywords: pituitary neuroendocrine tumors; VEGF; Treg; TAM; PD-1; PD-L1

1. Introduction

Pituitary neuroendocrine tumors (PitNETs) are common intracranial tumors that arise from the pituitary gland [1]. In recent years, the development of transnasal endoscopic surgery has improved the surgical outcomes in patients with PitNETs. However, PitNETs often invade into the surrounding cavernous sinus (CS), making them difficult to remove entirely. Although radiation therapy including gamma knife is performed for residual tumors [2], it is onerous to protect essential structures including the optic nerve and internal carotid artery around the sella turcica.

The vascular endothelial growth factor (VEGF)/VEGF receptor (VEGFR) signaling is a potent activator of angiogenesis that is known to correlate with disease progression and hemorrhage in PitNETs [3,4]. The difference in the status of VEGF/VEGFR signaling remains controversial. Niveiro et al. [3] demonstrated that the lowest protein level of VEGF-A was detected in prolactin-secreting

PitNETs and the highest levels were detected in non-functional PitNETs (NF-PitNETs). In contrast, Cristina et al. [4] demonstrated that higher expressions of VEGF-A and VEGFR1 were observed in prolactin-secreting PitNETs than in NF-PitNETs.

Recently, the significance of the programmed cell death-1 (PD-1)/programmed cell death ligand-1 (PD-L1) immune checkpoint system in various types of tumors has received attention [5,6]. Anti-PD-1 and PD-L1 antibodies exerted a highly potent effect in the inhibition of tumor growth in melanoma, non-small lung cancer, and kidney cancer [7,8]. Among immune cell types of note, M2 macrophages produce growth factors and anti-inflammatory cytokines to suppress the host immune response [9–11]. Tumor-associated macrophages (TAMs) typically behave as M2 macrophages in the tumor immune microenvironment to induce immunosuppression [12–14]. Regulatory T cells (Tregs) also exert immunosuppression, resulting in the failure of cancer immunotherapy [15,16]. High Foxp3(+) Tregs infiltration was significantly associated with shorter overall survival in most patients with solid tumors including melanomas and cervical, renal, and breast cancers [17]. VEGF-A plays a pivotal role in the development of these immunosuppressive microenvironments by inhibiting the maturation of dendritic cells and stimulating the proliferation of Tregs [18,19]. However, these immunosuppressive microenvironments have not been fully elucidated in PitNETs.

In the present study, VEGF-A/VEGFRs expressions, the tumor immune microenvironment, and their cross interaction were evaluated, leading to the development of novel treatment strategies for patients with NF-PitNETs.

2. Materials and Methods

This research was approved by the Institutional Review Board of our institute (Reference number: 20050002). Written informed consent was obtained from all patients.

2.1. Study Population

From April 2011 to October 2017, a total of 27 patients with newly diagnosed NF-PitNETs were analyzed in the present study. All patients received neurosurgical procedures, for mass reduction or diagnostic biopsy, and did not receive radiochemotherapy before the operations.

2.2. Immunohistochemical Analysis

Histopathological analyses were performed on 3 μm sections of formalin-fixed paraffin-embedded sections of 27 tumors from 27 patients with newly diagnosed NF-PitNETs that were determined on the basis of the hormonal status in the peripheral blood. NF-PitNETs are usually soft and easy to remove via aspiration. A small amount of tissue was used for pathology assessment. In the present study, a large size of tissue was selected because the multiple, most vascularized regions (hot spots) should be screened for regionally averaged positive cell counts. Mitotic activity was assessed using hematoxylin and eosin (H&E) staining. Immunohistochemistry was performed according to standard procedures [20]. After tissue sections were deparaffinized and rehydrated, antigen retrieval was performed in citrate buffer (Ki-67, p53, VEGFR1, CD34, Foxp3, CD163, CD3, CD4, and PD-1), or in Tris buffer (pH 9 for VEGF-A, VEGFR2, CD8, HIF-1α, and PD-L1) using microwave irradiation or autoclave (HIF-1α and PD-L1). The sections were blocked for 60 min in 2.5% horse serum (ImmPRESSTM Detection Systems, Vectorlabs, CA, USA). The sections were incubated overnight at 4 °C with anti-Ki-67 antibody (1:200, M7249, DAKO), anti-p53 monoclonal antibody (1:100, DO-7, DAKO), anti-VEGF-A antibody (1:200, JH121, Merck Millipore), anti-VEGFR1 antibody (1:200, AF321, R&D SYSTEMS), anti-VEGFR2 antibody (1:600, 55B11, Cell Signaling Technology), anti-CD34 antibody (1:100,°C F1604, Nichirei Biosciences Inc.), anti-Foxp3 antibody (1:100, ab54501, Abcam), anti-CD163 antibody (1:100, ab87099, Abcam), anti-CD3 antibody (1:100, ab5690, Abcam), anti-CD4 antibody (1:200, 1F6, Nichirei Bioscience Inc.), anti-CD8 antibody (1:50, ab17147, Abcam), anti-hypoxia-inducible factor-1α (HIF-1α) antibody (1:100, H-206, Santa Cruz Biotechnology), anti-PD-1 antibody (1:50, NAT105, Abcam), and anti-PD-L1 antibody (1:500, 28-8, Abcam), then incubated with anti-mouse, anti-rabbit, or anti-goat

Ig secondary antibody (ImmPRESSTM Detection Systems, Vectorlabs) for 60 min at room temperature. The products were visualized with a peroxidase-diaminobenzidine reaction.

For the assessment of Ki-67 index, manual counting of 1000 tumor cells was routinely done at a high-power field (HPF: ×40) [21]. The positivity of VEGF-A staining in the tumor cytoplasm or stroma was assessed as the following: ++, diffuse intense staining; +, diffuse faint staining; −, negative staining. The staining positivity of VEGFR1 and VEGFR2 on endothelial cells was assessed as the following: +, staining in vascular endothelial cells; −, negative staining. For the assessment of microvessel density (MVD), the tissue sections were screened at low-power fields (×4), and the three most vascularized regions (hot spots) were selected for each region. The counting of microvessels was performed on these regions at HPFs (×20, 0.95 mm^2). HIF-1α expression was assessed as the following: ++, expression in >10% of tumor cells; +, expression in ≤10% of tumor cells; −, negative staining [22]. For the assessment of density of Foxp3, CD163, CD4, and CD8 (+) cells, the tissue sections were screened using each immunohistochemistry at the low-power fields (×4), and three hot spots were selected. Counting of the positive cells was performed in these areas at the HPFs (×40, 0.47 mm^2). PD-L1 expression was assessed as the following: 3+, expression in ≥50% of tumor cells; 2+, expression in ≥5% and <50% of tumor cells; 1+, expression in ≥1% and <5% of tumor cells; 0, expression in <1% of tumor cells [23]. Both histopathological reviewing and scoring were independently performed with blinded clinical information by three authors (MS, RT, and YM).

The specificity of immunohistochemistry was checked using negative and positive controls. For negative controls, paraffin sections were incubated with non-immune mouse, rabbit, and goat IgG at the same concentration used for each antibody. Sections from glioblastomas were used as the positive controls for each antibody (Figure S1).

2.3. Radiographical Analysis

The existence of CS invasion was evaluated by gadolinium (Gd)-enhanced T1-weighted images. We classified NF-PitNETs into two types: NF-PitNETs with CS invasion and NF-PitNETs without CS invasion. Cystic formation and hemorrhage components were evaluated using T1- or T2-weighted images. Tumor size was volumetrically measured via Gd-enhanced imaging, as previously described [20].

2.4. Statistical Analysis

Student's *t*-test was used for the quantitative analysis of Ki-67, mitotic count, Foxp 3, CD 163, PD-1, CD 4, and CD 8 (+) cells and the ratio of Foxp3 (+) cells to CD8 (+) cells in the CS (+) group and the CS (−) group. For the scores of VEGF-A, VEGFR1, VEGFR2, HIF-1α, and p53 the chi-squared test was used. PD-L1 expression on tumor cells was scored according to the percentage of PD-L1 positive cells (score 0–4). Therefore, nonparametric analysis of Mann-Whitney U-test was used to test the immunostaining raw scores of PD-L1 expression between the two groups, considering that the analytical immunohistochemistry scores were not normally distributed. All statistical analyses were performed using IBM SPSS statistics (IBM Corp., Armonk, NY, USA). A *p*-value of <0.05 was considered statistically significant.

3. Results

3.1. Patients' Characteristics

Characteristics of 27 patients with newly diagnosed NF-PitNETs are summarized in Table 1. The patients were categorized into a CS (+) group (n = 17) and a CS (−) group (n = 10) (Figure 1, Table 1). The average age of patients with NF-PitNETs exhibiting CS invasion was higher than in those without CS invasion (p = 0.0030). There was no significant difference in terms of sex in both groups (p = 0.45). Tumor volume was significantly higher in the CS (+) group than in the CS (−) group (p = 0.0011). However, some NF-PitNETs easily invade into the CS despite their small tumor size. There were no significant differences between the two groups in cystic formation ($p = 0.78$) and hemorrhagic component ($p = 0.89$).

Table 1. Patient characteristics and results.

	CS Invasion (+)	CS Invasion (−)	p Value
Number	17	10	-
Age (years old)	66.06 (37–85)	49.45 (32–76)	0.0030
Sex	Male: 6, Female: 11	Male: 5, Female: 5	0.45
Cystic formation	6	3	0.78
Hemorrhagic component	2	1	0.89
Tumor volume (cm^3)	27.75 ± 22.33	7.16 ± 7.23	0.0011
Ki-67 index	<1%: 17	<1%: 10	-
Mitotic count	0/10HPF: 13 1/10HPF: 3 2/10HPF: 1	0/10HPF: 9 1/10HPF: 1	0.38
p53 IHC positive	0	0	-
VEGF-A expression	++: 6 + or −: 11	++: 0 + or −: 10	0.033
VEGFR1 expression	+: 12 −: 5	+: 3 −: 7	0.040
CD163 expression	7.70 ± 10.9	2.60 ± 3.53	0.046

CS: cavernous sinus, IHC: immunohistochemistry, VEGF: vascular endothelial growth factor, VEGFR: vascular endothelial growth factor receptor.

3.2. Histological Analysis

No significant differences were observed in mitotic count between the two groups ($p = 0.38$) (Figure 1, Table 1). Ki-67 index was <1%, and p53 was immunonegative in all patients (Figure 1, Table 1).

3.3. Expressions of VEGF-Related Molecules and MVD

Expressions of VEGF-A and VEGFR1 were significantly higher in the CS (+) group than in the CS (−) group (VEGF-A: $p = 0.033$, VEGFR1: $p = 0.04$) (Figure 2). VEGFR2 expression showed no significant difference between the two groups ($p = 0.28$). VEGF-A and VEGFR1 were expressed on not only endothelial cells, but also on tumor cells. MVD showed no significant difference between the two groups ($p = 0.42$; Figure 2), and the average of all cases in both groups, 24.9/3HPF, was equivalent to that of other central nervous tumors with high vasculatures, previously described [19]. Expression of HIF-1α showed no significant difference between the two groups ($p = 0.88$; Figure 2).

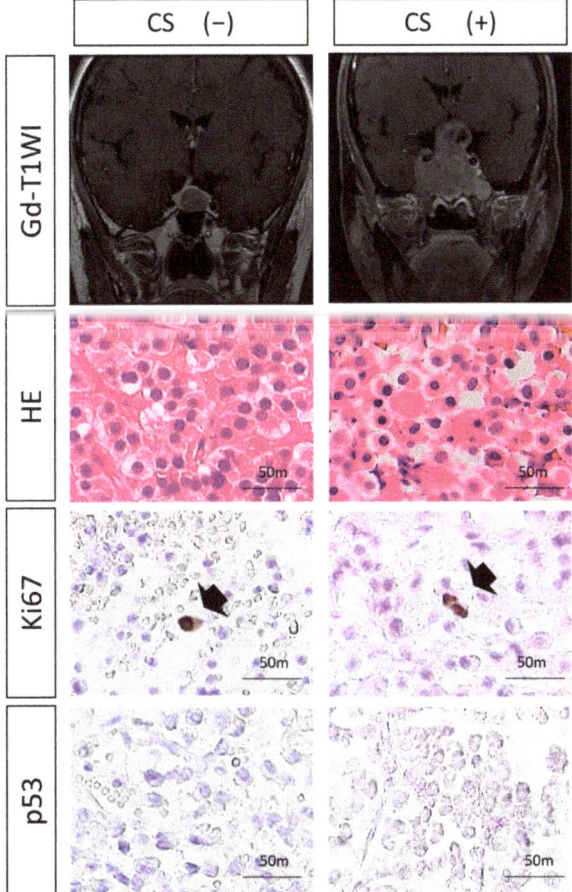

Figure 1. Analysis of classical histological atypical features for invasive non-functional pituitary neuroendocrine tumors (NF-PitNETs). The existence of CS invasion was evaluated by gadolinium (Gd)-enhanced T1-weighted images. There were no significant differences in Ki-67 and p53 expression or mitotic count between NF-PitNETs with CS invasion and NF-PitNETs without CS invasion (Ki-67 and mitotic count, student's t-test; p53, chi-squared test). Black arrow: tumor cell showing positive Ki-67 expression (Original magnification, ×20).

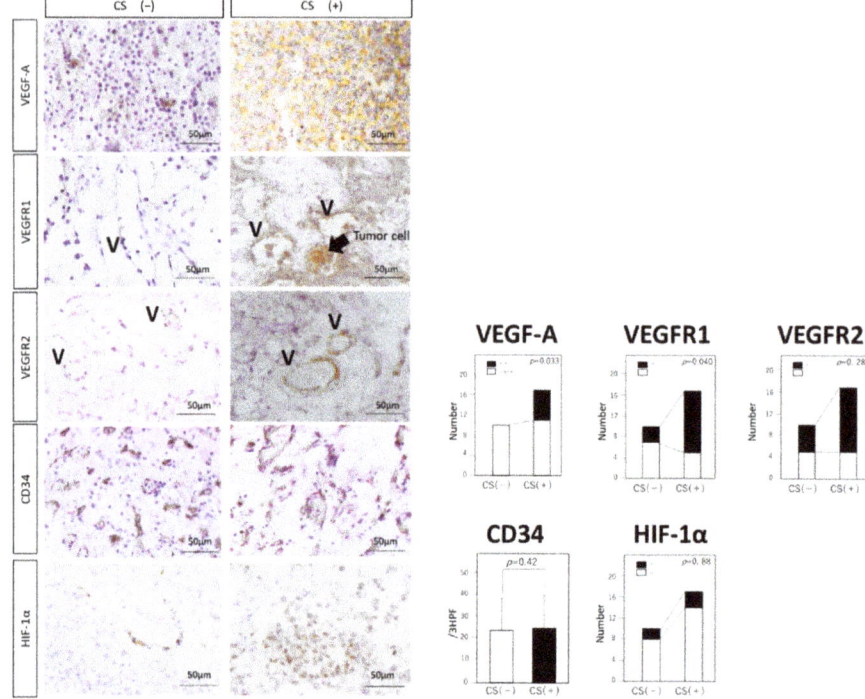

Figure 2. Expressions of VEGF-A related molecules in NF-PitNETs. Immunohistochemical analysis of VEGF-A, VEGFR1, VEGFR2, CD34, and HIF-1. Typical examples of each staining are shown in both groups. Black arrow: tumor cells showing positive VEGFR1 expression. V: vascular structure (original magnification, ×20). Statistical analysis of each staining is shown. Expressions of VEGF-A and VEGFR1 are significantly higher in the CS (+) group than in the CS (−) group (VEGF-A: $p = 0.033$, VEGFR1: $p = 0.040$). Expressions of VEGFR2 and HIF-1α do not reach statistical significance (VEGFR2: $p = 0.28$, HIF1-α: $p = 0.88$). MVD shows no significant difference between the two groups ($p = 0.42$). Data represent the mean ± standard error of mean (VEGF-A, VEGFR1, VEGFR2 and HIF-1α, chi-squared test; MVD, student's t-test).

3.4. Tumor-Infiltrating Immune Cells

The number of CD8 (+) lymphocytes tended to be higher in the CS (+) group than in the CS (−) group, but the difference is not statistically significant (10.81 vs. 2.9, $p = 0.052$; Figure 3). The number of CD4 (+) lymphocytes showed no significant difference between the two groups (6.94 vs. 4.89, $p = 0.28$; Figure 3). The number of immunosuppressive CD163 (+) cells was significantly higher in the CS (+) group than in the CS (−) group (7.7 vs. 2.6, $p = 0.046$; Figure 4). Although the number of immunosuppressive Foxp3 (+) cells showed no significant difference between the two groups (0.5 vs. 0.4, $p = 0.39$; Figure 4), Foxp3/CD8 ratio was significantly higher in the CS (+) group than in the CS (−) group (25.87 vs. 7.25, $p = 0.0059$; Figure 4).

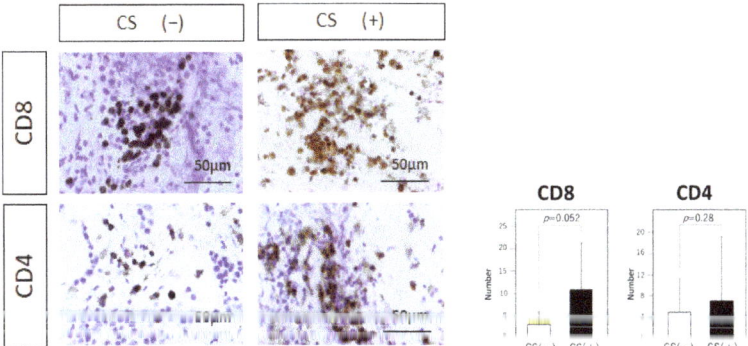

Figure 3. Analysis of tumor-infiltrating lymphocytes. Immunohistochemical analysis of CD8 and CD4 (Original magnification, ×20). Typical examples of each staining are shown in both groups. Statistical analysis of each staining is shown. The number of CD8 (+) lymphocytes tends to be higher in the CS (+) group than in the CS (−) group, but the difference is not statistically significant ($p = 0.052$). The number of CD4 (+) lymphocytes shows no significant difference between the two groups ($p = 0.28$). Data represent the mean ± standard error of mean (CD4 and CD8, student's t-test).

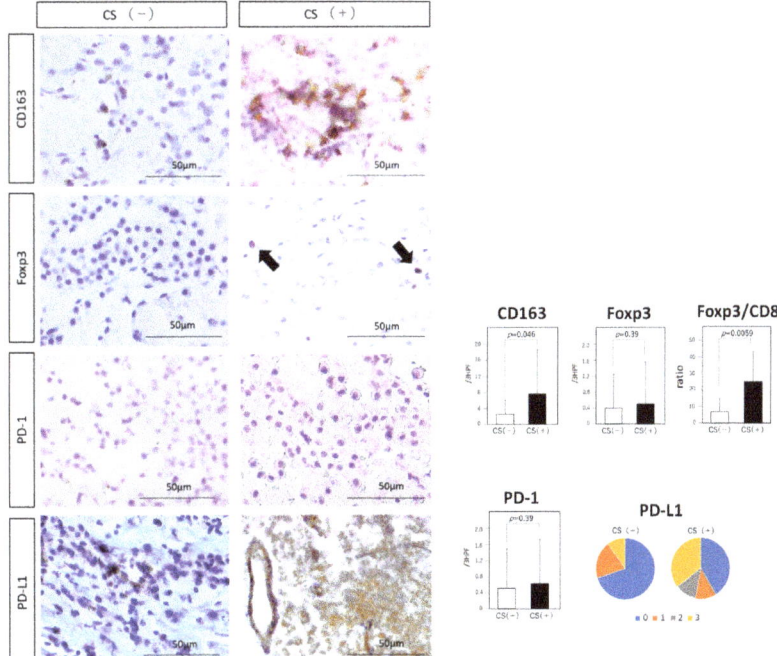

Figure 4. Analysis of immunosuppressive cells and immune checkpoint molecules. Immunohistochemical analysis of CD163, Foxp3, PD-1, and PD-L1 (Original magnification, ×20). Typical examples of each staining are shown in both groups. Black arrow: tumor cell showing positive Foxp3 expression. The number of CD163 (+) tumor-associated macrophages (TAMs) and Foxp3/CD8 ratio are significantly higher in the CS (+) group than in the CS (−) group (CD163: $p = 0.046$, Foxp3/CD8: $p = 0.0059$). The score of PD-L1 tends to be higher in the CS (+) group than in the CS (−) group ($p = 0.050$). Expressions of Foxp3 and PD-1 do not reach statistical significance (Foxp3: $p = 0.39$, PD-1: $p = 0.39$). Data represent the mean ± standard error of mean (CD163, Foxp3, PD-1 and Foxp3/CD8 ratio, student's t-test; PD-L1, Mann-Whitney U test).

3.5. Immune Checkpoint Molecules

The expression of PD-L1 was observed on cell membrane and in the cytoplasm of tumor cells (Figure 4). The endothelial cells were also occasionally immunopositive for PD-L1. In the CS (+) group, the PD-L1 score was 2 or 3 in eight patients, and 0 or 1 in nine of the 17 patients. In contrast, in the CS (−) group, the PD-L1 score was 2 or 3 in one patient, and 0 or 2 in nine of the 10 patients. The score tended to be higher in the CS (+) group than in the CS (−) group, but the difference is not statistically significant ($p = 0.050$; Figure 4). There were no significant differences in PD-1 (+) cells between the two groups (0.61 vs. 0.50, $p = 0.39$).

4. Discussion

CS invasion is a commonly demonstrated aggressive behavior exhibited by PitNETs [24–26], and this property has been recommended to describe aggressive PitNETs in the revised 2017 World Health Organization (WHO) classification [1]. Recently, Rutkowski et al. [27] re-emphasized the importance of classical histological characteristics. They demonstrated that mitotic activity, extensive p53 staining, and Ki-67 index were associated with poor prognosis [27]. However, in the present study, these classical histological characteristics did not show a correlation with CS invasion.

In contrast, our data suggested that VEGF-A/VEGFR1 expressions could be associated with CS invasion. The relationship between the expressions of VEGF-A/VEGFR1 and the prognosis of PitNETs has been previously discussed [28,29]. VEGF-A and VEGFR1 are known to contribute to the tumor cell growth of PitNETs [28,30,31]. Some studies have demonstrated that VEGFR2 is widely expressed in NF-PitNETs, with aggressive behavior such as suprasellar extension in NF-PitNETs [3,32]. MVD, characterized by CD31 immunopositivity and VEGF-A expression, reflected poor prognosis of NF-PitNETs [4]. Our findings corroborate with the findings of these studies. Importantly, VEGF-A and VEGFR1 were expressed on not only endothelial cells, but also on tumor cells, which have been previously confirmed using PitNETs cell line HP75 [33,34]. Tumor cells expressing VEGFR1 themselves release VEGF-A, and an autocrine regulatory function for VEGF in tumor growth in PitNETs is plausible.

Xiao et al. demonstrated rapid and hemorrhagic transformation in PitNETs via the HIF-1α hypoxic signaling pathway [35]. Interestingly, there was no significant correlation in the expression levels of HIF-1α and VEGF mRNA in PitNETs, although VEGF-A is mainly induced by HIF-1α [35]. RSUME, a small RWD-domain containing protein, was reported to play an important role in tumor neovascularization by regulating VEGF-A production in PitNETs [36–39]. The lack of correlation between VEGF-A and HIF-1α observed in the present study is in accordance with previous observations [35]. It is noteworthy that Barbagallo et al. [40] demonstrated that circSMARCA5, which acts as circular RNA for the splicing factor Serine and Arginine Rich Splicing Factor 1 SRSF1 in glioblastomas, is an upstream regulator of VEGF-A. Other regulators, such as circSMARCA5, might be involved in the VEGF-A expression of PitNETs.

Other aggressive characteristics, such as cystic change, were previously correlated with upregulated VEGF-A [29]. However, controversy exists over the relationship between hemorrhagic change and VEGF-A expression [29,41]. VEGF-A was not associated with cystic or hemorrhagic change in the present study. The cause for the discrepancy in the status of cystic and hemorrhage change between previous relevant studies and this study remains unclear. It could be attributed to the small sample size, highly heterogeneous PitNETs, and the difference between the analytical methods of immunohistochemistry and quantitative analysis (RT-PCR and western blot). Although VEGF-A is widely considered as a marker of poor prognosis in PitNETs, Takada et al. could not find significant correlations between vascularity and other clinical and endocrinological parameters, suggesting that angiogenesis is not essential for growth or invasiveness of PitNETs [42]. Further analysis using a large number of patients might elucidate the role of VEGF-A in PitNETs.

There is a lack of studies related to the tumor microenvironment of PitNETs. PD-L1 RNA and protein expression were significantly increased in recurrent functioning (growth hormone and prolactin-expressing) PitNETs compared with in NF-PitNETs (null cell and silent gonadotroph). Tumor infiltrating CD8 (+) lymphocytes were positively correlated with increased PD-L1 expression [43,44]. In the present study, most NF-PitNETs without CS invasion showed low PD-L1 expression score and low CD8 (+) lymphocyte count, which was compatible with previous studies [43,44]. However, some NF-PitNETs with CS invasion demonstrated a high PD-L1 expression score and a high number of CD8 (+) lymphocyte counts. Interestingly, PD-1/PD-L1 expressions are known to be associated with VEGF-A exposure [45,46].

Tumor size in NF-PitNETs is positively correlated with the number of CD68+ macrophages [47]. Macrophages express different functional programs in response to microenvironmental signals, which is defined as M1/M2 polarization [48]. CD68 antigen is expressed on both M1 and M2 macrophages, and CD163 is a specific marker for M2 macrophages [48]. Although the number of CD163 + M2 macrophages (TAMs) was not associated with the tumor volume, TAMs were associated with CS invasion in the present study. TAMs produce matrix metalloproteinase (MMP)-9 [48] that might promote the invasive behavior of PitNETs. Furthermore, VEGF-A is known to promote the immunosuppressive microenvironment [49], as well as the migration and differentiation of TAMs from immature myeloid cells [50,51].

Upregulation of VEGF-A induces VEGFR-2-expressing Tregs and also promotes their recruitment to the tumor microenvironment via over-expression of chemokine—chemokine ligand 28 by tumor cells [52]. Foxp3/CD8 ratio are known to correlate with the immunosuppressive microenvironment [46,53]. In the present study, the Foxp3/CD8 ratio was strongly associated with CS invasion, which might serve as a new biomarker of invasive NF-PitNETs.

The results obtained in the present study suggest that VEGF-A/VEGFR1 expression can be a treatment target. Blocking VEGF-A can regulate immunosuppressive cells such as TAMs. However, PitNETS with high PD-L1 expression deserve special attention as they correlate to poor outcomes of certain chemo- and immunotherapies [45,54–57].

A limitation of this study was the paucity of the number of patients. Other invasive markers such as MMP-9 and -14 were previously correlated with the hemorrhage and invasive behavior of PitNETs [41,58]. Future studies should analyze the role of these MMPs in a large number of patients to confirm the findings of this study. In addition, NF-PitNETs are morphologically heterogeneous. The new classification by WHO in 2017 was based on hormone immunohistochemistry and pituitary transcription factors. Although gonadotroph adenoma is the most common subtype among non-functional adenomas [1,59], some cases with thyroid stimulating hormone (TSH), growth hormone (GH), adrenocorticotropic hormone (ACTH), or prolactin (PRL) stainings behave as silent adenomas with no secretion [1]. The relationship between VEGF/VEGFR signaling, tumor microenvironment, and the above-mentioned hormonal and transcriptional characteristics should be investigated in future studies.

5. Conclusions

The high expressions of VEGF-A and VEGFR1 were observed in NF-PitNETs with CS invasion. Immunosuppressive microenvironments including TAMs and immune checkpoint molecules, which are induced by VEGF-A, were also associated with NF-PitNETs with CS invasion.

Supplementary Materials: The following are available online at http://www.mdpi.com/2077-0383/8/5/695/s1, Figure S1: Positive controls for each antibody.

Author Contributions: The following statements should be used "conceptualization, M.S., R.T. and M.T.; methodology, M.S., H.T., T.M., K.K., Y.M., and R.T.; software, M.S., and K.K.; validation, R.T., M.T., and K.Y.; formal analysis, M.S., K.K., and R.T.; investigation, M.S., H.T., T.M., M.T., K.K., Y.M., and R.T.; data curation, M.S., K.K., and R.T.; writing—original draft preparation, M.S., H.T., M.T., and R.T.; writing—review and editing, K.K., M.T., and K.Y.; visualization, M.S., and R.T.; supervision, K.Y.; funding acquisition, M.T.

Funding: This work was supported in part by grants from the Japan Society for the Promotion of Science (JSPS) (17H04306 and 18K19622 and to MT).

Conflicts of Interest: The authors declare no conflicts of interest.

References

1. Mete, O.; Lopes, M.B. Overview of the 2017 WHO Classification of Pituitary Tumors. *Endocr. Pathol.* **2017**, *28*, 228–243. [CrossRef] [PubMed]
2. Albano, L.; Losa, M.; Nadin, F.; Barzaghi, L.R.; Parisi, V.; del Vecchio, A.; Bolognesi, A.; Mortini, P. Safety and efficacy of multisession gamma knife radiosurgery for residual or recurrent pituitary adenomas. *Endocrine* **2019**. [CrossRef]
3. Niveiro, M.; Aranda, F.; Peiró, G.; Alenda, C.; Picó, A. Immunohistochemical analysis of tumor angiogenic factors in human pituitary adenomas. *Hum. Pathol.* **2005**, *36*, 1090–1095. [CrossRef]
4. Cristina, C.; Perez-Millan, M.; Luque, G.; Dulce, RA.; Sevlever, G.; Berner, S.I.; Becu-Villalobos, D. VEGF and CD31 association in pituitary adenomas. *Endocr. Pathol.* **2010**, *21*, 154–160. [CrossRef]
5. Iwai, Y.; Okazaki, T.; Nishimura, H.; Kawasaki, A.; Yagita, H.; Honjo, T. Microanatomical localization of PD-1 in human tonsils. *Immunol. Lett.* **2002**, *83*, 215–220. [CrossRef]
6. Iwai, Y.; Terawaki, S.; Ikegawa, M.; Okazaki, T.; Honjo, T. PD-1 inhibits antiviral immunity at the effector phase in the liver. *J. Exp. Med.* **2003**, *198*, 39–50. [CrossRef]
7. Butte, M.J.; Keir, M.E.; Phamduy, T.B.; Sharpe, A.H.; Freeman, G.J. Programmed death-1 ligand 1 interacts specifically with the B7-1 costimulatory molecule to inhibit T cell responses. *Immunity* **2007**, *27*, 111–122. [CrossRef] [PubMed]
8. Rizvi, N.A.; Hellmann, M.D.; Snyder, A.; Kvistborg, P.; Makarov, V.; Havel, J.J.; Lee, W.; Yuan, J.; Wong, P.; Ho, T.S.; et al. Cancer immunology. Mutational landscape determines sensitivity to PD-1 blockade in non-small cell lung cancer. *Science* **2015**, *348*, 124–128. [CrossRef]
9. Allavena, P.; Sica, A.; Garlanda, C.; Mantovani, A. The Yin-Yang of tumor-associated macrophages in neoplastic progression and immune surveillance. *Immunol. Rev.* **2008**, *222*, 155–161. [CrossRef]
10. Charo, I.F. Macrophage polarization and insulin resistance: PPARgamma in control. *Cell Metab.* **2007**, *6*, 96–98. [CrossRef]
11. Medzhitov, R.; Horng, T. Transcriptional control of the inflammatory response. *Nat. Rev. Immunol.* **2009**, *9*, 692–703. [CrossRef] [PubMed]
12. Franklin, R.A.; Liao, W.; Sarkar, A.; Kim, M.V.; Bivona, M.R.; Liu, K.; Pamer, E.G.; Li, M.O. The cellular and molecular origin of tumor-associated macrophages. *Science* **2014**, *344*, 921–925. [CrossRef] [PubMed]
13. Qian, B.Z.; Li, J.; Zhang, H.; Kitamura, T.; Zhang, J.; Campion, L.R.; Kaiser, E.A.; Snyder, L.A.; Pollard, J.W. CCL2 recruits inflammatory monocytes to facilitate breast-tumour metastasis. *Nature* **2011**, *475*, 222–225. [CrossRef]
14. Shand, F.H.; Ueha, S.; Otsuji, M.; Koid, S.S.; Shichino, S.; Tsukui, T.; Kosugi-Kanaya, M.; Abe, J.; Tomura, M.; Ziogas, J.; et al. Tracking of intertissue migration reveals the origins of tumor-infiltrating monocytes. *Proc. Natl. Acad. Sci. USA* **2014**, *111*, 7771–7776. [CrossRef]
15. Wang, H.Y.; Lee, D.A.; Peng, G.; Guo, Z.; Li, Y.; Kiniwa, Y.; Shevach, E.M.; Wang, R.F. Tumor-specific human CD4+ regulatory T cells and their ligands: Implications for immunotherapy. *Immunity* **2004**, *20*, 107–118. [CrossRef]
16. Vignali, D.A.; Collison, L.W.; Workman, C.J. How regulatory T cells work. *Nat. Rev. Immunol.* **2008**, *8*, 523–532. [CrossRef] [PubMed]
17. Whiteside, T.L. The tumor microenvironment and its role in promoting tumor growth. *Oncogene* **2008**, *27*, 5904–5912. [CrossRef]
18. Gabrilovich, D.I.; Chen, H.L.; Girgis, K.R.; Cunningham, H.T.; Meny, G.M.; Nadaf, S.; Kavanaugh, D.; Carbone, D.P. Production of vascular endothelial growth factor by human tumors inhibits the functional maturation of dendritic cells. *Nat. Med.* **1996**, *2*, 1096–1103. [CrossRef]
19. Ohm, J.E.; Gabrilovich, D.I.; Sempowski, G.D.; Kisseleva, E.; Parman, K.S.; Nadaf, S.; Carbone, D.P. VEGF inhibits T-cell development and may contribute to tumor-induced immune suppression. *Blood* **2003**, *101*, 4878–4886. [CrossRef]
20. Tamura, R.; Ohara, K.; Sasaki, H.; Morimoto, Y.; Yoshida, K.; Toda, M. Histopathological vascular investigation of the peritumoral brain zone of glioblastomas. *J. Neurooncol.* **2018**, *136*, 233–241. [CrossRef]
21. Tamura, R.; Ohara, K.; Morimoto, Y.; Kosugi, K.; Oishi, Y.; Sato, M.; Yoshida, K.; Toda, M. PITX2 Expression in Non-functional Pituitary Neuroendocrine Tumor with Cavernous Sinus Invasion. *Endocr. Pathol.* **2019**, *22*. [CrossRef]

22. Tamura, R.; Tanaka, T.; Miyake, K.; Tabei, Y.; Ohara, K.; Sampetrean, O.; Kono, M.; Mizutani, K.; Yamamoto, Y.; Murayama, Y.; et al. Histopathological investigation of glioblastomas resected under bevacizumab treatment. *Oncotarget* **2016**, *7*, 52423–52435. [CrossRef]
23. Fehrenbacher, L.; Spira, A.; Ballinger, M.; Kowanetz, M.; Vansteenkiste, J.; Mazieres, J.; Park, K.; Smith, D.; Artal-Cortes, A.; Lewanski, C.; et al. Atezolizumab versus docetaxel for patients with previously treated non-small-cell lung cancer (POPLAR): A multicentre, open-label, phase 2 randomised controlled trial. *Lancet* **2016**, *387*, 1837–1846. [CrossRef]
24. Asa, S.L.; Casar-Borota, O.; Chanson, P.; Delgrange, E.; Earls, P.; Ezzat, S.; Grossman, A.; Ikeda, H.; Inoshita, N.; Karavitaki, N.; et al. From pituitary adenoma to pituitary neuroendocrine tumor (PitNET): An International Pituitary Pathology Club proposal. *Endocr. Relat. Cancer* **2017**, *24*, C5–C8. [CrossRef]
25. Rindi, G.; Klimstra, D.S.; Abedi-Ardekani, B.; Asa, S.L.; Bosman, F.T.; Brambilla, E.; Busam, K.J.; de Krijger, R.R.; Dietel, M.; El-Naggar, A.K.; et al. A common classification framework for neuroendocrine neoplasms: An International Agency for Research on Cancer (IARC) and World Health Organization (WHO) expert consensus proposal. *Mod. Pathol.* **2018**, *31*, 1770–1786. [CrossRef]
26. Delellis, R.A.; Lloyd, R.V.; Heitz, P.U.; Eng, C. Pathology and Genetics of Tumors of Endocrine Organs. In *WHO Classification of Tumors*, 3rd ed.; World Health Organization: Geneva, Switzerland, 2004; Volume 8.
27. Rutkowski, M.J.; Alward, R.M.; Chen, R.; Wagner, J.; Jahangiri, A.; Southwell, D.G.; Kunwar, S.; Blevins, L.; Lee, H.; Aghi, M.K. Atypical pituitary adenoma: A clinicopathologic case series. *J. Neurosurg.* **2018**, *128*, 1058–1065. [CrossRef] [PubMed]
28. McCabe, C.J.; Boelaert, K.; Tannahill, L.A.; Heaney, A.P.; Stratford, A.L.; Khaira, J.S.; Hussain, S.; Sheppard, M.C.; Franklyn, J.A.; Gittoes, N.J. Vascular endothelial growth factor, its receptor KDR/Flk-1, and pituitary tumor transforming gene in pituitary tumors. *J. Clin. Endocrinol. Metab.* **2002**, *87*, 4238–4244. [CrossRef]
29. Fukui, S.; Otani, N.; Nawashiro, H.; Yano, A.; Nomura, N.; Tokumaru, A.M.; Miyazawa, T.; Ohnuki, A.; Tsuzuki, N.; Katoh, H.; et al. The association of the expression of vascular endothelial growth factor with the cystic component and haemorrhage in pituitary adenoma. *J. Clin. Neurosci.* **2003**, *10*, 320–324. [CrossRef]
30. Shimoda, Y.; Ogawa, Y.; Watanabe, M.; Tominaga, T. Clinicopathological investigation of vascular endothelial growth factor and von Hippel-Lindau gene-related protein expression in immunohistochemically negative pituitary adenoma—Possible involvement in tumor aggressiveness. *Endocr. Res.* **2013**, *38*, 242–250. [CrossRef]
31. Lee, S.W.; Lee, J.E.; Yoo, C.Y.; Ko, M.S.; Park, C.S.; Yang, S.H. NRP-1 expression is strongly associated with the progression of pituitary adenomas. *Oncol. Rep.* **2014**, *32*, 1537–1542. [CrossRef]
32. Sánchez-Ortiga, R.; Sánchez-Tejada, L.; Moreno-Perez, O.; Riesgo, P.; Niveiro, M.; Picó Alfonso, A.M. Over-expression of vascular endothelial growth factor in pituitary adenomas is associated with extrasellar growth and recurrence. *Pituitary* **2013**, *16*, 370–377. [CrossRef]
33. Horiguchi, H.; Jin, L.; Ruebel, K.H.; Scheithauer, B.W.; Lloyd, R.V. Regulation of VEGF-A, VEGFR-I, thrombospondin-1, -2, and -3 expression in a human pituitary cell line (HP75) by TGFbeta1, bFGF, and EGF. *Endocrine* **2004**, *24*, 141–146. [CrossRef]
34. Onofri, C.; Theodoropoulou, M.; Losa, M.; Uhl, E.; Lange, M.; Arzt, E.; Stalla, G.K.; Renner, U. Localization of vascular endothelial growth factor (VEGF) receptors in normal and adenomatous pituitaries: Detection of a non-endothelial function of VEGF in pituitary tumours. *J Endocrinol.* **2006**, *191*, 249–261. [CrossRef]
35. Xiao, Z.; Liu, Q.; Zhao, B.; Wu, J.; Lei, T. Hypoxia induces hemorrhagic transformation in pituitary adenomas via the HIF-1α signaling pathway. *Oncol. Rep.* **2011**, *26*, 1457–1464. [CrossRef]
36. Kim, K.; Yoshida, D.; Teramoto, A. Expression of hypoxia-inducible factor 1alpha and vascular endothelial growth factor in pituitary adenomas. *Endocr. Pathol.* **2005**, *16*, 115–121. [PubMed]
37. Shan, B.; Gerez, J.; Haedo, M.; Fuertes, M.; Theodoropoulou, M.; Buchfelder, M.; Losa, M.; Stalla, G.K.; Arzt, E.; Renner, U. RSUME is implicated in HIF-1-induced VEGF-A production in pituitary tumour cells. *Endocr. Relat. Cancer* **2012**, *19*, 13–27. [CrossRef] [PubMed]
38. Fowkes, R.C.; Vlotides, G. Hypoxia-induced VEGF production 'RSUMEs' in pituitary adenomas. *Endocr. Relat. Cancer* **2012**, *19*, C1–C5. [CrossRef] [PubMed]
39. He, W.; Huang, L.; Shen, X.; Yang, Y.; Wang, D.; Yang, Y.; Zhu, X. Relationship between RSUME and HIF-1α/VEGF-A with invasion of pituitary adenoma. *Gene* **2017**, *603*, 54–60. [CrossRef] [PubMed]
40. Barbagallo, D.; Caponnetto, A.; Brex, D.; Mirabella, F.; Barbagallo, C.; Lauretta, G.; Morrone, A.; Certo, F.; Broggi, G.; Caltabiano, R.; et al. CircSMARCA5 Regulates VEGFA mRNA Splicing and Angiogenesis in Glioblastoma Multiforme Through the Binding of SRSF1. *Cancers* **2019**, *11*, 194. [CrossRef] [PubMed]

41. Xiao, Z.; Liu, Q.; Mao, F.; Wu, J.; Lei, T. TNF-α-induced VEGF and MMP-9 expression promotes hemorrhagic transformation in pituitary adenomas. *Int. J. Mol. Sci.* **2011**, *12*, 4165–4179. [CrossRef]
42. Takada, K.; Yamada, S.; Teramoto, A. Correlation between tumor vascularity and clinical findings in patients with pituitary adenomas. *Endocr. Pathol.* **2004**, *15*, 131–139. [CrossRef]
43. Mei, Y.; Bi, W.L.; Greenwald, N.F.; Du, Z.; Agar, N.Y.; Kaiser, U.B.; Woodmansee, W.W.; Reardon, D.A.; Freeman, G.J.; Fecci, P.E.; et al. Increased expression of programmed death ligand 1 (PD-L1) in human pituitary tumors. *Oncotarget* **2016**, *7*, 76565–76576. [CrossRef]
44. Wang, P.F.; Wang, T.J.; Yang, Y.K.; Yao, K.; Li, Z.; Li, Y.M.; Yan, C.X. The expression profile of PD-L1 and CD8+ lymphocyte in pituitary adenomas indicating for immunotherapy. *J. Neurooncol.* **2018**, *139*, 89–95. [CrossRef]
45. Voron, T.; Colussi, O.; Marcheteau, E.; Pernot, S.; Nizard, M.; Pointet, A.L.; Latreche, S.; Bergaya, S.; Benhamouda, N.; Tanchot, C.; et al. VEGF-A modulates expression of inhibitory checkpoints on CD8+ T cells in tumors. *J. Exp. Med.* **2015**, *212*, 139–148. [CrossRef]
46. Tamura, R.; Tanaka, T.; Ohara, K.; Miyake, K.; Morimoto, Y.; Yamamoto, Y.; Kanai, R.; Akasaki, Y.; Murayama, Y.; Tamiya, T.; et al. Persistent restoration to the immunosupportive tumor microenvironment in glioblastoma by bevacizumab. *Cancer Sci.* **2019**, *110*, 499–508. [CrossRef]
47. Lu, J.Q.; Adam, B.; Jack, A.S.; Lam, A.; Broad, R.W.; Chik, C.L. Immune Cell Infiltrates in Pituitary Adenomas: More Macrophages in Larger Adenomas and More T Cells in Growth Hormone Adenomas. *Endocr. Pathol.* **2015**, *26*, 263–272. [CrossRef]
48. Tamura, R.; Tanaka, T.; Yamamoto, Y.; Akasaki, Y.; Sasaki, H. Dual role of macrophage in tumor immunity. *Immunotherapy* **2018**, *10*, 899–909. [CrossRef]
49. Wang, M.; Zhao, J.; Zhang, L.; Wei, F.; Lian, Y.; Wu, Y.; Gong, Z.; Zhang, S.; Zhou, J.; Cao, K.; et al. Role of tumor microenvironment in tumorigenesis. *J. Cancer* **2017**, *8*, 761–773. [CrossRef]
50. Quail, D.F.; Joyce, J.A. Microenvironmental regulation of tumor progression and metastasis. *Nat. Med.* **2013**, *19*, 1423–1437. [CrossRef]
51. Ott, P.A.; Hodi, F.S.; Buchbinder, E.I. Inhibition of Immune Checkpoints and Vascular Endothelial Growth Factor as Combination Therapy for Metastatic Melanoma: An Overview of Rationale, Preclinical Evidence, and Initial Clinical Data. *Front. Oncol.* **2015**, *5*, 202. [CrossRef]
52. Wada, J.; Yamasaki, A.; Nagai, S.; Yanai, K.; Fuchino, K.; Kameda, C.; Tanaka, H.; Koga, K.; Nakashima, H.; Nakamura, M.; et al. Regulatory T-cells are possible effect prediction markers of immunotherapy for cancer patients. *Anticancer Res.* **2008**, *28*, 2401–2408.
53. Takada, K.; Kashiwagi, S.; Goto, W.; Asano, Y.; Takahashi, K.; Takashima, T.; Tomita, S.; Ohsawa, M.; Hirakawa, K.; Ohira, M. Use of the tumor-infiltrating CD8 to FOXP3 lymphocyte ratio in predicting treatment responses to combination therapy with pertuzumab, trastuzumab, and docetaxel for advanced HER2-positive breast cancer. *J. Transl. Med.* **2018**, *16*, 86. [CrossRef]
54. Xue, S.; Hu, M.; Li, P.; Ma, J.; Xie, L.; Teng, F.; Zhu, Y.; Fan, B.; Mu, D.; Yu, J. Relationship between expression of PD-L1 and tumor angiogenesis, proliferation, and invasion in glioma. *Oncotarget* **2017**, *8*, 49702–49712. [CrossRef]
55. He, J.; Hu, Y.; Hu, M.; Li, B. Development of PD-1/PD-L1 Pathway in Tumor Immune Microenvironment and Treatment for Non-Small Cell Lung Cancer. *Sci. Rep.* **2015**, *5*, 13110. [CrossRef]
56. Jacobs, J.F.; Idema, A.J.; Bol, K.F.; Nierkens, S.; Grauer, O.M.; Wesseling, P.; Grotenhuis, J.A.; Hoogerbrugge, P.M.; de Vries, I.J.; Adema, G.J. Regulatory T cells and the PD-L1/PD-1 pathway mediate immune suppression in malignant human brain tumors. *Neuro-Oncology* **2009**, *11*, 394–402. [CrossRef]
57. Kalathil, S.G.; Lugade, A.A.; Miller, A.; Iyer, R.; Thanavala, Y. PD-1+ and Foxp3+ T cell reduction correlates with survival of HCC patients after sorafenib therapy. *JCI Insight* **2016**, *21*, 1. [CrossRef]
58. Hui, P.; Xu, X.; Xu, L.; Hui, G.; Wu, S.; Lan, Q. Expression of MMP14 in invasive pituitary adenomas: Relationship to invasion and angiogenesis. *Int. J. Clin. Exp. Pathol.* **2015**, *8*, 3556–3567. [PubMed]
59. Manojlovic-Gacic, E.; Engström, B.E.; Casar-Borota, O. Histopathological classification of non-functioning pituitary neuroendocrine tumors. *Pituitary* **2018**, *21*, 119–129. [CrossRef]

© 2019 by the authors. Licensee MDPI, Basel, Switzerland. This article is an open access article distributed under the terms and conditions of the Creative Commons Attribution (CC BY) license (http://creativecommons.org/licenses/by/4.0/).

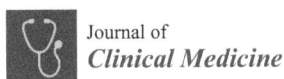

Article

A Pilot Study of Vaccine Therapy with Multiple Glioma Oncoantigen/Glioma Angiogenesis-Associated Antigen Peptides for Patients with Recurrent/Progressive High-Grade Glioma

Ryogo Kikuchi [1,2], Ryo Ueda [2,3], Katsuya Saito [4], Shunsuke Shibao [4], Hideaki Nagashima [2], Ryota Tamura [2], Yukina Morimoto [2], Hikaru Sasaki [2], Shinobu Noji [5], Yutaka Kawakami [5], Kazunari Yoshida [2] and Masahiro Toda [2,*]

1. Department of Neurosurgery, Hiratsuka City Hospital, Hiratsuka, Kanagawa 254-0019, Japan; fi020084@yahoo.co.jp
2. Department of Neurosurgery, Keio University School of Medicine, Shinjuku, Tokyo 160-8587, Japan; ueda.ryo@gmail.com (R.U.); 032m2068@gmail.com (H.N.); moltobello-r-610@hotmail.co.jp (R.T.); yukinaxnashiko@yahoo.co.jp (Y.M.); hsasaki@a5.keio.jp (H.S.); Kazrmky@keio.jp (K.Y.)
3. Department of Neurosurgery, Kawasaki Municipal Hospital, Kawasaki, Kanagawa 210-0013, Japan
4. Department of Neurosurgery, Ashikaga Red Cross Hospital, Ashikaga, Tochigi 326-0843, Japan; csrbb415@yahoo.co.jp (K.S.); pochisuke616@mac.com (S.S.)
5. Division of Cellular Signaling, Institute for Advanced Medical Research, Keio University School of Medicine, Shinjku, Tokyo 160-8587, Japan; snoji@keio.jp (S.N.); yutakawa@keio.jp (Y.K.)
* Correspondence: todam@keio.jp; Tel.: +81-3-3353-1211; Fax: +81-3-3358-0479

Received: 11 January 2019; Accepted: 14 February 2019; Published: 20 February 2019

Abstract: High-grade gliomas (HGGs) carry a dismal prognosis despite current treatments. We previously confirmed the safety and immunogenicity of a vaccine treatment targeting tumor angiogenesis with synthetic peptides, for vascular endothelial growth factor receptor (VEGFR) epitopes in recurrent HGG patients. In this study, we evaluated a novel vaccine therapy targeting not only tumor vasculature but also tumor cells, using multiple glioma oncoantigen (GOA)/glioma angiogenesis-associated antigen (GAAA) peptides in HLA-A2402+ recurrent/progressive HGG patients. The vaccine included peptide epitopes from four GOAs (LY6K, DEPDC1, KIF20A, and FOXM1) and two GAAAs (VEGFR1 and VEGFR2). Ten patients received subcutaneous vaccinations. The primary endpoint was the safety of the treatment. T-lymphocyte responses against GOA/GAAA epitopes and treatment response were evaluated secondarily. The treatment was well tolerated without any severe systemic adverse events. The vaccinations induced immunoreactivity to at least three vaccine-targeted GOA/GAAA in all six evaluable patients. The median overall survival time in all patients was 9.2 months. Five achieved progression-free status lasting at least six months. Two recurrent glioblastoma patients demonstrated stable disease. One patient with anaplastic oligoastrocytoma achieved complete response nine months after the vaccination. Taken together, this regimen was well tolerated and induced robust GOA/GAAA-specific T-lymphocyte responses in recurrent/progressive HGG patients.

Keywords: vaccine therapy; oncoantigen; tumor associate antigen; tumor angiogenesis; high-grade glioma

---

1. Introduction

High-grade gliomas (HGGs) carry a dismal prognosis despite current treatments [1–4]. Options are particularly limited for patients with recurrent HGGs so new therapies are needed. Cancer vaccines are promising in this regard, designed to induce systemic immunity against antigens overexpressed by tumor cells and other components in the tumor microenvironment. Pilot clinical trials by us and others have exhibited the safety and potential efficacy of cytotoxic T lymphocyte (CTL) epitope peptide-based vaccinations for patients with HGGs [5–11].

Although cancer vaccines have been anticipated as a promising modality to treat cancer, recent reports indicated several mechanisms in tumor tissues that protect cancer cells from immune attacks [12]. For example, the limitation of the antitumor effects of CTLs was explained by inter- and intra-tumoral heterogeneity; a subset of tumor cells revealed downregulation, or loss of expression of human leukocyte antigen (HLA), or targeted antigen proteins [13,14]. To overcome the suppression of CTL antitumor effects, which occur due to tumor cell heterogeneity, we previously focused on a peptide vaccine targeting the tumor vasculature in the tumor microenvironment and demonstrated the safety and immunogenicity of vaccination with synthetic peptides for vascular endothelial growth factor receptor (VEGFR) epitopes in recurrent HGG patients [11].

Targeting of multiple glioma antigen epitopes also helps to address the issue of inter- and intra-tumoral heterogeneity of glioma cells. Furthermore, "oncoantigens" are ideal targets for a cancer vaccine [15–21] as they are essential for cell growth, and the probability of immune escape of cancer cells by reducing or lacking these proteins is expected to be low [22]. Therefore, this clinical trial was based on the use of HLA-A2402–restricted CTL epitopes derived from four glioma oncoantigens (GOAs) that we and others observed to be highly expressed in HGGs [23–26]: Lymphocyte antigen 6 family member K (LY6K), DEP domain containing 1 (DEPDC1), kinesin family member 20A (KIF20A), and forkhead box M1 (FOXM1)—in addition to two glioma angiogenesis-associated antigen (GAAAs): VEGFR1 and VEGFR2 [27,28].

To the best of our knowledge, this is the first study to evaluate a glioma vaccine therapy targeting tumor vasculature, as well as tumor cells with multiple glioma antigen epitope peptides derived from glioma cell-expressed oncoantigens and glioma angiogenesis factors. The primary objectives were to assess the tolerability of this regimen and its ability to induce GOA/GAAA epitope-specific immune responses.

2. Materials and Methods

The study protocol was approved by the institutional ethics committee (#20130294).

2.1. Vaccine Therapy Design

This study was a non-randomized, open label clinical trial with cocktail peptide vaccines for recurrent/progressive HGGs. The primary endpoint of this study was the safety of the peptide vaccine treatment. Secondary endpoints were the GOA/GAAA epitope–specific immune responses and the therapeutic outcome of patients treated with this vaccine.

2.2. Patient Eligibility

As we wished to focus on safety and immunoreactivity to the antigens in this vaccine treatment, we enrolled patients with recurrent/progressive HGG (World Health Organization (WHO) grade III/IV glioma) including, but not limited to, glioblastoma (grade IV glioma) from April 2014 to November 2016 at Keio University Hospital (Tokyo, Japan)—resulting in a somewhat heterogenous patient cohort.

Inclusion criteria were as follows: (1) histological diagnosis of supratentorial HGG (World Health Organization (WHO) grade III or IV according to the 2007 WHO criteria) without multiple lesions or leptomeningeal dissemination; (2) patients were informed about their diagnosis; (3) HLA-A*2402-positive status; (4) age between 16 and 79 years; (5) Eastern Cooperative Oncology performance status 0–2; (6) completion of standard treatment (surgical therapy + radiation therapy + temozolomide); (7) four-week interval from last chemotherapy or radiotherapy; (8) adequate bone-marrow, cardiac, pulmonary, and hepatic and renal functions including neutrophil $\geq 1000/\mu L$, platelet count $\geq 50,000/\mu L$, hemoglobin ≥ 8 g/dL, plasma aspartate aminotransferase and alanine aminotransferase levels ≤ 4 times the normal limit, plasma bilirubin levels ≤ 1.5 times the normal limit, plasma albumin levels ≥2.5 g/dL, and plasma creatinine levels ≤2.0 mg/dL; (9) life expectancy >3 months; (10) signature confirming informed consent. Exclusion criteria were as follows: (1) uncontrollable infection; (2) the presence of another serious disease such as uncontrolled diabetes, hepatic disorder, cardiac disease, hemorrhage/bleeding; (3) total parenteral nutrition; (4) multiple cancers; (5) myelodysplastic syndrome (MDS), MDS/myeloproliferative disease (MPD) and MPD; (6) allogenic hematopoietic stem cell transplantation; (7) severe immunological disorders (autoimmune disease, immunosuppression); (8) anaphylaxis to synthetic peptides; (9) concurrent treatment with steroids or immunosuppressive agents; (10) pregnant or breast-feeding women; (11) severe mental disorder; (12) unhealed wound; (13) decision of unsuitability by the principal investigator or the physician in charge.

2.3. Peptides

The peptide vaccine included HLA-A2402-restricted epitopes for four GOAs (LY6K, DEPDC1, KIF20A, and FOXM1) and two GAAAs (VEGFR1 and VEGFR2). These peptide epitopes have been previously identified and evaluated for safety and potent immunogenicity in various cancer patients: a VEGFR1-derived peptide (VEGFR1-1084; SYGVLLWEI) [29], a VEGFR2-derived peptide (VEGFR2-169; RFVPDGNRI) [30], a LY6K-derived peptide (LY6K-177; RYCNLEGPPI) [31], a DEPDC1-derived peptide (DEPDC1-294; EYYELFVNI) [16], a KIF20A-derived peptide (KIF20A-66; KVYLRVRPLL) [32], and a FOXM1-derived peptide (FOXM1-262; IYTWIEDHF) [33]. All GMP-grade peptides were synthesized by the American Peptide Company (Sunnyvale, CA, USA) according to a standard solid-phase synthesis method and purified by reversed-phase high-performance liquid chromatography (HPLC). The purity (>90%) and identity of the peptides were determined by analytical HPLC and mass spectrometry analysis, respectively.

2.4. Vaccine Preparation and Treatment Protocol

One milligram of each peptide was emulsified in incomplete Freund's adjuvant (Montanide ISA-51VG; SEPPIC, Paris, France) and administered subcutaneously close to an axillary or inguinal lymph node, eight times weekly. Patients demonstrating no clinical or radiological progression without adverse events had the option of continuing to receive vaccinations at 2-week intervals, for up to 8 months after the initial vaccination.

2.5. Radiologic Response Monitoring and Other Clinical Endpoints

Tumor size was assessed at weeks 9, 17, 25, and 33, then every 3 months thereafter using magnetic resonance imaging (MRI) with contrast enhancement. Response was evaluated by the Response Evaluation Criteria in Solid Tumors [34] and Immunotherapy Response Assessment in Neuro-Oncology [35] by gadolinium-enhanced T1 weighted images on the basis of the appearance of the pretreatment MRI. Overall survival (OS) was defined by the interval from initial vaccination to date of death. MRI was used to evaluate tumor progression over time.

2.6. Toxicity Assessment

Toxicity was assessed based on the common terminology criteria for adverse effects version 4.0. Toxicity was defined as toxicity of grade 4 or greater.

2.7. CTL Responses to Peptide Stimulation

To evaluate the specific CD8+ T-cell response, an enzyme-linked immunosorbent spot (ELISPOT) assay was performed in six cases using a procedure reported in a prior study [11].

Table 1. Patient characteristics

Case No.	Age (Years)	Sex	Diagnosis	Tumor Size (mm)	Operation	Radiotherapy	Chemotherapy	IDH1 Mutation	1p/19q Codeletion	MGMT Methylation
1	17	M	GB	32.5 × 29.5 × 32.5	2	60 Gy	TMZ, ICE	WT	(−)	(−)
2	38	M	HGG	20.6 × 11.7 × 16.6	0	60 Gy + SRT30 Gy	TMZ	NT	NT	NT
3	38	M	GB with oligo	No enhanced lesion *	2	60 Gy	TMZ	WT	NT	(−)
4	66	F	GB	18.0 × 11.5 × 20.0	1	60 Gy	TMZ, BEV	NT	NT	NT
5	46	F	sGB	48.0 × 25.0 × 48.8	5	GK, 60 Gy	TMZ, IFNb, BEV	NT	NT	NT
6	33	F	AOA	12.0 × 8.5 × 18.0	4	60 Gy	TMZ	R132H	(−)	(±)
7	72	M	OA rec	33.0 × 20.5 × 23.7	1	60 Gy	TMZ, BEV	WT	(−)	(−)
8	36	F	sGB	16.0 × 13.0 × 18.6	2	60 Gy	TMZ, BEV	R132H	(−)	(−)
9	27	F	sGB	30.2 × 24.1 × 28.6	1	SRT	TMZ, BEV	R132H	(−)	(+)
10	67	F	GB	23.3 × 12.1 × 17.5	2	60 Gy	TMZ	WT	(−)	(±)

AOA, anaplastic oligoastrocytoma; BEV, bevacizumab; F, female; GB, glioblastoma; GB with oligo, glioblastoma with oligodendroglial component; GK, gamma knife; HGG, high grade glioma; ICE, ifosfamide, carboplatin, and etoposide; IDH, Isocitrate dehydrogenase; IFNb, interferon beta; M, male; MGMT, O-6-methylguanine-DNA-methyl-transferase; NT, not tested; OA rec, recurrent oligoastrocytoma; sGB, secondary glioblastoma; SRT, stereotactic radiotherapy; TMZ, temozolomide; WT, wild type. * This patient was enrolled after complete recurrent tumor removal.

2.8. Statistical Analysis

Statistical analyses were performed using SPSS 24.0 software (IBM, Chicago, IL, USA). OS curves were estimated using Kaplan–Meier methodology. Statistical analyses were performed with the log-rank test and differences were considered statistically significant at $p < 0.05$.

3. Results

3.1. Demographics and Clinical Characteristics

A total of 10 patients—who were found to be HLA-A2402 positive by DNA typing of HLA genomic variations—were enrolled in this study. Three patients were initially treated in other hospitals. Mean age was 44 years old (range, 17–72). Mean follow-up was 16.2 months (range, 3.6–38.1). Seven of the 10 patients were diagnosed with glioblastoma. Table 1 shows the characteristics of the 10 enrolled patients.

3.2. Toxicity

No severe adverse events associated with the vaccine were observed. During the vaccination therapy, skin flare (grade 1) was shown in one patient and induration (grade 1) was shown in five patients at the injection site. Wound infection (grade 2) and herpes zoster (grade 2) were each found in a single patient during the observation period and were considered to be unrelated to the vaccination.

3.3. CTL Response

CTL responses were analyzed in six evaluable patients, as shown in Table 2. All six patients showed specific CTL responses to at least three vaccine-targeted GOA/GAAA epitopes.

Table 2. Cytotoxic T lymphocyte (CTL) responses to target antigens.

Case No.	Vaccination	LY6K	FOXM1	DEPDC1	KIF20A	VEGFR1	VEGFR2	Positive Control
1	before	−	+	+	+	+	−	+++
	2 weeks after	+++	+++	+++	+	+	−	+++
2	before	−	−	+	+	−	−	+++
	2 weeks after	+++	+++	+++	+	−	−	+++
3	before	−	−	NT	NT	−	NT	+++
	2 weeks after	+	+++	+	−	+	NT	+++
4	before	−	+	+	−	−	+	+++
	2 weeks after	+++	+++	+++	+	−	+	+++
5	before	−	+	−	−	−	−	+++
	2 weeks after	+++	+++	+++	+	+	+++	+++
6	before	−	+	−	−	−	−	+++
	2 weeks after	+++	+++	+++	+	+	+++	+++

NT, not tested.

3.4. Clinical Outcomes

Although the primary goal of this study was to provide an analysis of safety and immunoreactivity, preliminary outcome data were obtained (Table 3 and Figure 1). Patients received a mean of 14.2 (range, 8–26) peptide vaccinations. One patient achieved partial response (PR), two patients demonstrated stable disease, and six patients revealed progressive disease 6 months after the first vaccination (Table 3). Patient 7 was removed from the study due to rapid tumor progression. Patients 3, 6, and 10 remain progression-free at 18, 38, and 11 months, respectively, after the first vaccination. Among these patients, Patient 6 achieved compete response (CR) 9 months after the first vaccination. These results indicate the preliminary efficacy of this treatment.

Table 3. Clinical results of 10 enrolled patients.

Case No.	Frequency of Vaccination	Period of Vaccination (mo)	Evaluation after 3 Months	Evaluation after 6 Months	PFS (mo)	OS (mo)
1	18	6.2	PD	PD	6.3	8.9
2	11	6.7	PD	PD	6.8	18.9
3	26	21.0	SD	SD	18.2	34.3
4	12	4.8	PD	PD	4.9	9.1
5	8	1.6	PD	PD	1.7	8.1
6	20	37.5	PR	PR *	38.1	38.1
7	8	1.6	PD	Dead	1.9	3.6
8	11	4.6	SD	PD	4.7	7.7
9	10	2.1	PD	PD	2.9	9.4
10	18	10.8	SD	SD	11.0	23.6

Mo, months; OS, overall survival; PD, progressive disease; PFS, progression-free survival; PR, partial response; SD, stable disease. * Complete response was achieved after 9 months.

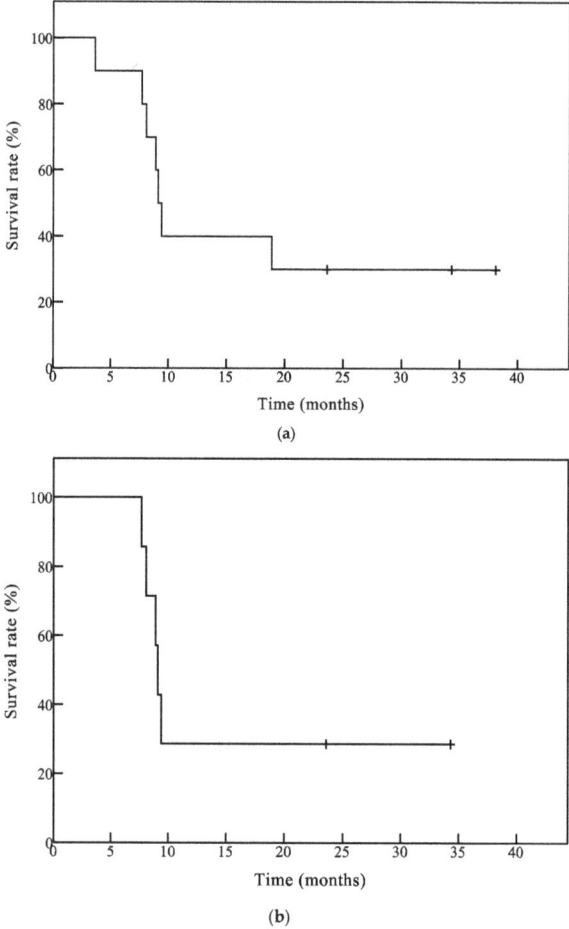

Figure 1. Survival analysis of patients by the Kaplan–Meier method. (**a**) Overall survival (OS) curve of all patients (n = 10). The median OS time (mOS) of all patients was 9.2 months and 1-year OS was 44.4%; (**b**) OS curve of glioblastoma (GB) patients (n = 7). The mOS was 9.1 months and 1-year OS was 33.3% in GB patients.

The Kaplan–Meier curves for overall survival in all 10 patients and seven glioblastoma (GB) patients are shown in Figure 1a,b, respectively. The median overall survival time (mOS) in all patients and GB patients was 9.2 months and 9.1 months, respectively. One-year OS was 44.4% for all patients and 33.3% for GB patients, respectively.

Five patients were treated with bevacizumab before registration. In this group, 1-year OS was 0% and mOS was 8.6 months. Otherwise, in GB patients who had not received bevacizumab before registration, mOS was 23.6 months. Our findings suggest that the GB patients who did not receive bevacizumab had a longer survival period than those treated with bevacizumab following a combination of chemotherapy and/or radiotherapy, but no significant differences in OS were observed—likely due to the small sample numbers.

3.5. A Case of CR following Peptide Vaccination

Patient 6 was a 33-year-old female diagnosed with diffuse astrocytoma (grade 2) four years prior. Her tumor was enlarged and removed twice, followed by treatment with TMZ and radiation therapy for the preceding 12 months. The pathological diagnosis was anaplastic oligoastrocytoma (grade 3, MGMT unmethylated, IDH mutant and no 1p19q codeletion). However, her tumor recurred and could not be removed as it was located in a functional area (Figure 2a). She was thus enrolled in our study. Her tumor decreased in size three months after vaccine initiation and disappeared nine months after enrollment (Figure 2b,c). Thirty-eight months after the initiation of peptide vaccination, the patient remains free of tumor recurrence.

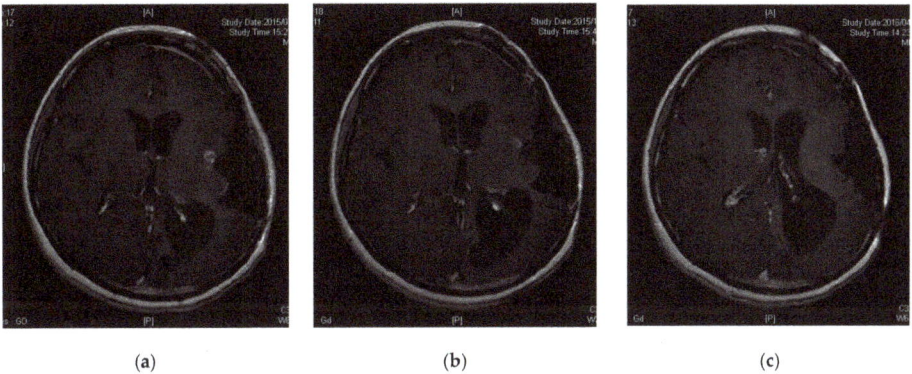

Figure 2. Contrast-enhanced magnetic resonance images of Patient 6. (**a**) Tumor had recurred in a functional area; (**b**) tumor was decreased 3 months after enrollment; (**c**) tumor disappeared 9 months after enrollment.

4. Discussion

This is the first clinical evaluation of peptide-based vaccine therapy, targeting glioma cells as well as glioma neovascular endothelial cells, using multiple GOA/GAAA-derived epitopes for recurrent/progressive HGG. Our findings demonstrate tolerability and immunoreactivity to GOAs/GAAAs, as well as the preliminary efficacy of this treatment.

The population was very small and not homogeneous in this study. However, this was a pilot study to assess safety and immunoreactivity to the antigens, which allowed us to assess the tolerability and immune response regardless of patient characteristics.

The peptide epitopes included in this vaccine treatment were derived from six proteins known as GOAs or GAAAs [23–28]. ELISPOT data demonstrated that all evaluable vaccinated patients mounted an immune response against at least three of the target antigens, supporting the use of such epitopes in glioma vaccine regimens. ELISPOT data also showed that CTLs specific for three oncoantigens, DEPDC1, FOXM1, and LY6K were frequently observed in peripheral blood mononuclear cells from the vaccinated patients—indicating that these oncoantigens are highly immunogenic in advanced HGG patients. To evaluate if the induced CTLs contributed to reduction of tumor cells or tumor vascular endothelial cells in the microenvironment, further immunohistochemical analyses of tumor tissues obtained from vaccinated patients or blood flow analyses that can detect hypoperfusion peri-/intra-tumorally are warranted.

Although this was a pilot study focusing on safety and immunoreactivity to the antigens, we also evaluated treatment response in the vaccinated patients. In this study, the mOS in all patients and GB patients was 9.2 months and 9.1 months, respectively. Our median survival results are comparable to, but do not exceed those reported in the literature by previous clinical studies of glioma vaccines [9,10] and various combination regimens of chemotherapy and/or radiotherapy for recurrent GB patients [36–39]. This may be reflected in immune tolerance or a hostile immune status mediated by regulatory T-cell populations or tumor-secreted immunosuppressive factors in immunocompromised patients with recurrent HGG. Previous studies have demonstrated that anti-VEGF agents, such as bevacizumab, inhibit proliferation of immunosuppressive cells, such as regulatory T-cells and myeloid derived suppressor cells [40–42]—suggesting that VEGF-VEGFR pathway blockade could restore and improve antitumor immune responses. Nevertheless, the HGG patients who did not receive bevacizumab had a longer survival period than the patients treated with bevacizumab following a combination of chemotherapy and/or radiotherapy, although the sample size was relatively small (Figure 3). These results suggest that such approaches may be most effective if applied early in treatment, particularly in patients likely to have a robust immunity, such as the patients who have not yet received any chemotherapy or radiation therapy. In fact, cancer vaccines often need more time to elicit beneficial immune responses that demonstrate biological activity, which is shown by the occurrence of delayed vaccine effects.

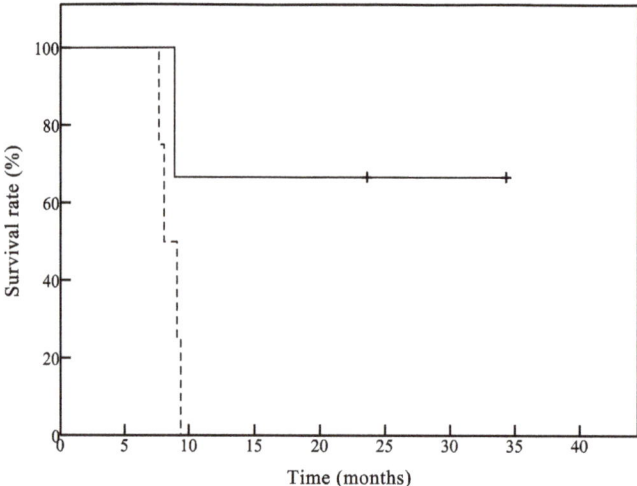

Figure 3. Overall survival of glioblastoma patients with or without bevacizumab. The median overall survival time (mOS) was 23.6 months in three patients that did not receive bevacizumab before enrollment (solid line). The mOS was 8.6 months in four patients treated with bevacizumab before enrollment (dotted line).

One HGG patient (Patient 6) experienced objective clinical tumor regression (response rate of this vaccine treatment was 10%). Furthermore, it is noteworthy that this patient exhibited PR at week six and CR at week nine. CTLs specific for all six antigens were strongly induced in the patients, suggesting that this CTL response might contribute to the observable effect.

As biological features of HGGs in children are different from those that arise in adults [43,44], it is necessary to discuss the cases of children specifically. Our heterogenous patient cohort included a 17 year-old patient, whose OS was 8.9 months after enrollment. This vaccine therapy could not extend OS significantly, but could safely induce CTLs specific for three oncoantigens in this patient, suggesting that this vaccine therapy theoretically has the potential to exert an antitumor effect for pediatric HGGs expressing target antigens. Therefore, immunoreactivity to antigens and clinical efficacy of this regimen for children with HGGs will be assessed in a future study.

In summary, we performed a pilot study for HLA-A2402+ patients with recurrent/progressive HGGs to assess the safety, feasibility, and immunoreactivity of the peptide-based vaccine targeting GOAs and GAAAs. The safety and immunogenicity of this vaccine therapy was verified. The data suggest that this vaccine treatment may show preliminary evidence of clinical responses. However, a future study of this vaccine in combination with standard treatment for newly-diagnosed HGGs as well as immune-checkpoint blockade therapies, is required to improve the efficacy of glioma vaccine therapy.

Author Contributions: Conceptualization, R.U. and M.T.; formal analysis, R.K. and S.N.; investigation, R.K., K.S., S.S., H.N., R.T., Y.M., H.S., and M.T.; resources, S.N., Y.K., and K.Y.; data curation, R.K.; writing—original draft preparation, R.K.; writing—review and editing, R.U. and M.T.; visualization, R.K.; supervision, Y.K. and K.Y.; project administration, M.T.; funding acquisition, R.K., R.U., and M.T.

Funding: This research was supported by the Japan Society for the Promotion of Science Grants-in-Aid for Young Scientists (B), Grant Number 17K16661.

Acknowledgments: We thank Yuko Aikawa and Tomoko Muraki (Department of Neurosurgery, Keio University School of Medicine) for their technical assistance. We also thank Gillian Campbell, PhD, from Edanz Group (www.edanzediting.com/ac) for editing a draft of this manuscript.

Conflicts of Interest: The authors declare no conflict of interest.

References

1. Stupp, R.; Mason, W.P.; van den Bent, M.J.; Weller, M.; Fisher, B.; Taphoorn, M.J.B.; Belanger, K.; Brandes, A.A.; Marosi, C.; Bogdahn, U.; et al. Radiotherapy plus concomitant and adjuvant temozolomide for glioblastoma. *N. Engl. J. Med.* **2005**, *352*, 987–996. [CrossRef] [PubMed]
2. Chinot, O.L.; Wick, W.; Mason, W.; Henriksson, R.; Saran, F.; Nishikawa, R.; Carpentier, A.F.; Hoang-Xuan, K.; Kavan, P.; Cernea, D.; et al. Bevacizumab plus radiotherapy-temozolomide for newly diagnosed glioblastoma. *N. Engl. J. Med.* **2014**, *370*, 709–722. [CrossRef] [PubMed]
3. Gilbert, M.R.; Dignam, J.J.; Armstrong, T.S.; Wefel, J.S.; Blumenthal, D.T.; Vogelbaum, M.A.; Colman, H.; Chakravarti, A.; Pugh, S.L.; Won, M.; et al. A randomized trial of bevacizumab for newly diagnosed glioblastoma. *N. Engl. J. Med.* **2014**, *370*, 699–708. [CrossRef] [PubMed]
4. Stupp, R.; Wong, E.T.; Kanner, A.A.; Steinberg, D.; Engelhard, H.; Heidecke, V.; Kirson, E.D.; Taillibert, S.; Liebermann, F.; Dbalý, V.; et al. NovoTTF-100A versus physician's choice chemotherapy in recurrent glioblastoma: A randomised phase III trial of a novel treatment modality. *Eur. J. Cancer* **2012**, *48*, 2192–2202. [CrossRef] [PubMed]
5. Sampson, J.H.; Heimberger, A.B.; Archer, G.E.; Aldape, K.D.; Friedman, A.H.; Friedman, H.S.; Gilbert, M.R.; Herndon, J.E.; McLendon, R.E.; Mitchell, D.A.; et al. Immunologic escape after prolonged progression-free survival with epidermal growth factor receptor variant III peptide vaccination in patients with newly diagnosed glioblastoma. *J. Clin. Oncol.* **2010**, *28*, 4722–4729. [CrossRef] [PubMed]
6. Pollack, I.F.; Jakacki, R.I.; Butterfield, L.H.; Hamilton, R.L.; Panigrahy, A.; Potter, D.M.; Connelly, A.K.; Dibridge, S.A.; Whiteside, T.L.; Okada, H. Antigen-specific immune responses and clinical outcome after vaccination with glioma-associated antigen peptides and polyinosinic-polycytidylic acid stabilized by lysine and carboxymethylcellulose in children with newly diagnosed malignant brainstem and nonbrainstem gliomas. *J. Clin. Oncol.* **2014**, *32*, 2050–2058. [CrossRef] [PubMed]

7. Okada, H.; Butterfield, L.H.; Hamilton, R.L.; Hoji, A.; Sakaki, M.; Ahn, B.J.; Kohanbash, G.; Drappatz, J.; Engh, J.; Amankulor, N.; et al. Induction of robust type-I CD8+ T-cell responses in WHO grade 2 low-grade glioma patients receiving peptide-based vaccines in combination with poly-ICLC. *Clin. Cancer Res.* **2015**, *21*, 286–294. [CrossRef] [PubMed]
8. Rampling, R.; Peoples, S.; Mulholland, P.J.; James, A.; Al-Salihi, O.; Twelves, C.J.; McBain, C.; Jefferies, S.; Jackson, A.; Stewart, W.; et al. A Cancer Research UK First Time in Human Phase I Trial of IMA950 (Novel Multipeptide Therapeutic Vaccine) in Patients with Newly Diagnosed Glioblastoma. *Clin. Cancer Res.* **2016**, *22*, 4776–4785. [CrossRef]
9. Terasaki, M.; Shibui, S.; Narita, Y.; Fujimaki, T.; Aoki, T.; Kajiwara, K.; Sawamura, Y.; Kurisu, K.; Mineta, T.; Yamada, A.; et al. Phase I trial of a personalized peptide vaccine for patients positive for human leukocyte antigen–A24 with recurrent or progressive glioblastoma multiforme. *J. Clin. Oncol.* **2011**, *29*, 337–344. [CrossRef]
10. Izumoto, S.; Tsuboi, A.; Oka, Y.; Suzuki, T.; Hashiba, T.; Kagawa, N.; Hashimoto, N.; Maruno, M.; Elisseeva, O.A.; Shirakata, T.; et al. Phase II clinical trial of Wilms tumor 1 peptide vaccination for patients with recurrent glioblastoma multiforme. *J. Neurosurg.* **2008**, *108*, 963–971. [CrossRef]
11. Shibao, S.; Ueda, R.; Saito, K.; Kikuchi, R.; Nagashima, H.; Kojima, A.; Kagami, H.; Pareira, E.S.; Sasaki, H.; Noji, S.; et al. A pilot study of peptide vaccines for VEGF receptor 1 and 2 in patients with recurrent/progressive high grade glioma. *Oncotarget* **2018**, *9*, 21569–21579. [CrossRef] [PubMed]
12. Rosenberg, S.A.; Yang, J.C.; Restifo, N.P. Cancer immunotherapy: moving beyond current vaccines. *Nat. Med.* **2004**, *10*, 909–915. [CrossRef] [PubMed]
13. Ryschich, E.; Nötzel, T.; Hinz, U.; Autschbach, F.; Ferguson, J.; Simon, I.; Weitz, J.; Fröhlich, B.; Klar, E.; Büchler, M.W.; et al. Control of T-cell-mediated immune response by HLA class I in human pancreatic carcinoma. *Clin. Cancer Res.* **2005**, *11*, 498–504. [CrossRef] [PubMed]
14. Khong, H.T.; Restifo, N.P. Natural selection of tumor variants in the generation of "tumor escape" phenotypes. *Nat. Immunol.* **2002**, *3*, 999–1005. [CrossRef] [PubMed]
15. Ishikawa, H.; Imano, M.; Shiraishi, O.; Yasuda, A. Phase I clinical trial of vaccination with LY6K-derived peptide in patients with advanced gastric cancer. *Gastric Cancer* **2013**. [CrossRef] [PubMed]
16. Obara, W.; Ohsawa, R.; Kanehira, M.; Takata, R.; Tsunoda, T.; Yoshida, K.; Takeda, K.; Katagiri, T.; Nakamura, Y.; Fujioka, T. Cancer peptide vaccine therapy developed from oncoantigens identified through genome-wide expression profile analysis for bladder cancer. *Jpn. J. Clin. Oncol.* **2012**, *42*, 591–600. [CrossRef] [PubMed]
17. Iwahashi, M.; Katsuda, M.; Nakamori, M.; Nakamura, M.; Naka, T.; Ojima, T.; Iida, T.; Yamaue, H. Vaccination with peptides derived from cancer-testis antigens in combination with CpG-7909 elicits strong specific CD8+ T cell response in patients with metastatic esophageal squamous cell carcinoma. *Cancer Sci.* **2010**, *101*, 2510–2517. [CrossRef]
18. Suzuki, H.; Fukuhara, M.; Yamaura, T.; Mutoh, S.; Okabe, N.; Yaginuma, H.; Hasegawa, T.; Yonechi, A.; Osugi, J.; Hoshino, M.; et al. Multiple therapeutic peptide vaccines consisting of combined novel cancer testis antigens and anti-angiogenic peptides for patients with non-small cell lung cancer. *J. Transl. Med.* **2013**, *11*, 97. [CrossRef]
19. Kono, K.; Iinuma, H.; Akutsu, Y.; Tanaka, H.; Hayashi, N.; Uchikado, Y.; Noguchi, T.; Fujii, H.; Okinaka, K.; Fukushima, R.; et al. Multicenter, phase II clinical trial of cancer vaccination for advanced esophageal cancer with three peptides derived from novel cancer-testis antigens. *J. Transl. Med.* **2012**, *10*, 141. [CrossRef] [PubMed]
20. Inoue, K.; Sugiura, F.; Kogita, A.; Yoshioka, Y.; Sukegawa, Y.; Hida, J.; Okuno, K. Clinical trial of a seven-peptide vaccine and tegafur-uracil/leucovorin as combination therapy for advanced colorectal cancer. *Gan Kagaku Ryoho* **2014**, *41*, 1276–1279.
21. Yoshitake, Y.; Fukuma, D.; Yuno, A.; Hirayama, M.; Nakayama, H.; Tanaka, T.; Nagata, M.; Takamune, Y.; Kawahara, K.; Nakagawa, Y.; et al. Phase II clinical trial of multiple peptide vaccination for advanced head and neck cancer patients revealed induction of immune responses and improved OS. *Clin. Cancer Res.* **2015**, *21*, 312–321. [CrossRef] [PubMed]
22. Lollini, P.; Cavallo, F.; Nanni, P.; Forni, G. Vaccines for tumour prevention. *Nat. Rev. Cancer* **2006**, *6*, 204–216. [CrossRef] [PubMed]

23. Zhang, N.; Wei, P.; Gong, A.; Chiu, W.; Lee, H.; Colman, H.; Huang, H.; Xue, J.; Liu, M.; Wang, Y.; et al. FoxM1 promotes β-catenin nuclear localization and controls Wnt target-gene expression and glioma tumorigenesis. *Cancer Cell* **2011**, *20*, 427–442. [CrossRef] [PubMed]
24. Kikuchi, R.; Sampetrean, O.; Saya, H.; Yoshida, K.; Toda, M. Functional analysis of the DEPDC1 oncoantigen in malignant glioma and brain tumor initiating cells. *J. Neurooncol.* **2017**, *133*, 297–307. [CrossRef] [PubMed]
25. Joshi, K.; Banasavadi-Siddegowda, Y.; Mo, X.; Kim, S.H.; Mao, P.; Kig, C.; Nardini, D.; Sobol, R.W.; Chow, L.M.L.; Kornblum, H.I.; et al. MELK-dependent FOXM1 phosphorylation is essential for proliferation of glioma stem cells. *Stem Cells* **2013**, *31*, 1051–1063. [CrossRef] [PubMed]
26. Saito, K.; Ohta, S.; Kawakami, Y.; Yoshida, K.; Toda, M. Functional analysis of KIF20A, a potential immunotherapeutic target for glioma. *J. Neurooncol.* **2017**, *132*, 63–74. [CrossRef] [PubMed]
27. Plate, K.H.; Risau, W. Angiogenesis in malignant gliomas. *Glia* **1995**, *15*, 339–347. [CrossRef]
28. Plate, K.H.; Breier, G.; Weich, H.A.; Mennel, H.D.; Risau, W. Vascular endothelial growth factor and glioma angiogenesis: coordinate induction of VEGF receptors, distribution of VEGF protein and possible in vivo regulatory mechanisms. *Int. J. Cancer* **1994**, *59*, 520–529. [CrossRef]
29. Ishizaki, H.; Tsunoda, T.; Wada, S.; Yamauchi, M.; Shibuya, M.; Tahara, H. Inhibition of tumor growth with antiangiogenic cancer vaccine using epitope peptides derived from human vascular endothelial growth factor receptor 1. *Clin. Cancer Res.* **2006**, *12*, 5841–5849. [CrossRef]
30. Wada, S.; Tsunoda, T.; Baba, T.; Primus, F.J.; Kuwano, H.; Shibuya, M.; Tahara, H. Rationale for antiangiogenic cancer therapy with vaccination using epitope peptides derived from human vascular endothelial growth factor receptor 2. *Cancer Res.* **2005**, *65*, 4939–4946. [CrossRef]
31. Suda, T.; Tsunoda, T.; Daigo, Y.; Nakamura, Y.; Tahara, H. Identification of human leukocyte antigen-A24-restricted epitope peptides derived from gene products upregulated in lung and esophageal cancers as novel targets for immunotherapy. *Cancer Sci.* **2007**, *98*, 1803–1808. [CrossRef] [PubMed]
32. Osawa, R.; Tsunoda, T.; Yoshimura, S.; Watanabe, T.; Miyazawa, M.; Tani, M.; Takeda, K.; Nakagawa, H.; Nakamura, Y.; Yamaue, H. Identification of HLA-A24-restricted novel T cell epitope peptides derived from P-cadherin and kinesin family member 20A. *J. Biomed. Biotechnol.* **2012**, *2012*. [CrossRef] [PubMed]
33. Yokomine, K.; Senju, S.; Nakatsura, T.; Irie, A.; Hayashida, Y.; Ikuta, Y.; Harao, M.; Imai, K.; Baba, H.; Iwase, H.; et al. The forkhead box M1 transcription factor as a candidate of target for anti-cancer immunotherapy. *Int. J. Cancer* **2010**, *126*, 2153–2163. [CrossRef] [PubMed]
34. Eisenhauer, E.A.; Therasse, P.; Bogaerts, J.; Schwartz, L.H.; Sargent, D.; Ford, R.; Dancey, J.; Arbuck, S.; Gwyther, S.; Mooney, M.; et al. New response evaluation criteria in solid tumours: Revised RECIST guideline (version 1.1). *Eur. J. Cancer* **2009**, *45*, 228–247. [CrossRef] [PubMed]
35. Okada, H.; Weller, M.; Huang, R.; Finocchiaro, G.; Gilbert, M.R.; Wick, W.; Ellingson, B.M.; Hashimoto, N.; Pollack, I.F.; Brandes, A.A.; et al. Immunotherapy response assessment in neuro-oncology: A report of the RANO working group. *Lancet Oncol.* **2015**, *16*, e534–e542. [CrossRef]
36. Wick, A.; Felsberg, J.; Steinbach, J.P.; Herrlinger, U.; Platten, M.; Blaschke, B.; Meyermann, R.; Reifenberger, G.; Weller, M.; Wick, W. Efficacy and tolerability of temozolomide in an alternating weekly regimen in patients with recurrent glioma. *J. Clin. Oncol.* **2007**, *25*, 3357–3361. [CrossRef] [PubMed]
37. Perry, J.R.; Bélanger, K.; Mason, W.P.; Fulton, D.; Kavan, P.; Easaw, J.; Shields, C.; Kirby, S.; Macdonald, D.R.; Eisenstat, D.D.; et al. Phase II trial of continuous dose-intense temozolomide in recurrent malignant glioma: RESCUE study. *J. Clin. Oncol.* **2010**, *28*, 2051–2057. [CrossRef]
38. Franceschi, E.; Cavallo, G.; Scopece, L.; Paioli, A.; Pession, A.; Magrini, E.; Conforti, R.; Palmerini, E.; Bartolini, S.; Rimondini, S.; et al. Phase II trial of carboplatin and etoposide for patients with recurrent high-grade glioma. *Br. J. Cancer* **2004**, *91*, 1038–1044. [CrossRef]
39. Nagane, M.; Nishikawa, R.; Narita, Y.; Kobayashi, H.; Takano, S.; Shinoura, N.; Aoki, T.; Sugiyama, K.; Kuratsu, J.; Muragaki, Y.; et al. Phase II study of single-agent bevacizumab in Japanese patients with recurrent malignant glioma. *Jpn. J. Clin. Oncol.* **2012**, *42*, 887–895. [CrossRef]
40. Terme, M.; Pernot, S.; Marcheteau, E.; Sandoval, F.; Benhamouda, N.; Colussi, O.; Dubreuil, O.; Carpentier, A.F.; Tartour, E.; Taieb, J. VEGFA-VEGFR pathway blockade inhibits tumor-induced regulatory T-cell proliferation in colorectal cancer. *Cancer Res.* **2013**, *73*, 539–549. [CrossRef]

41. Adotevi, O.; Pere, H.; Ravel, P.; Haicheur, N.; Badoual, C.; Merillon, N.; Medioni, J.; Peyrard, S.; Roncelin, S.; Verkarre, V.; et al. A decrease of regulatory T cells correlates with overall survival after sunitinib-based antiangiogenic therapy in metastatic renal cancer patients. *J. Immunother.* **2010**, *33*, 991–998. [CrossRef] [PubMed]
42. Du Four, S.; Maenhout, S.K.; Benteyn, D.; De Keersmaecker, B.; Duerinck, J.; Thielemans, K.; Neyns, B.; Aerts, J.L. Disease progression in recurrent glioblastoma patients treated with the VEGFR inhibitor axitinib is associated with increased regulatory T cell numbers and T cell exhaustion. *Cancer Immunol. Immunother.* **2016**, *65*, 727–740. [CrossRef] [PubMed]
43. Sturm, D.; Pfister, S.M.; Jones, D.T.W. Pediatric Gliomas: Current Concepts on Diagnosis, Biology, and Clinical Management. *J. Clin. Oncol.* **2017**, *35*, 2370–2377. [CrossRef] [PubMed]
44. Paugh, B.S.; Qu, C.; Jones, C.; Liu, Z.; Adamowicz-Brice, M.; Zhang, J.; Bax, D.A.; Coyle, B.; Barrow, J.; Hargrave, D.; et al. Integrated molecular genetic profiling of pediatric high-grade gliomas reveals key differences with the adult disease. *J. Clin. Oncol.* **2010**, *18*, 3061–3068. [CrossRef] [PubMed]

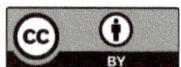

© 2019 by the authors. Licensee MDPI, Basel, Switzerland. This article is an open access article distributed under the terms and conditions of the Creative Commons Attribution (CC BY) license (http://creativecommons.org/licenses/by/4.0/).

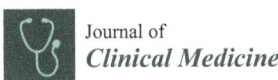

Review

The Inflammatory Milieu of Adamantinomatous Craniopharyngioma and Its Implications for Treatment

Ros Whelan [1,*], Eric Prince [1,2,3], Ahmed Gilani [4] and Todd Hankinson [1,2,3]

1. Department of Neurosurgery, University of Colorado Hospital, Aurora, CO 80045, USA; eric.prince@cuanschutz.edu (E.P.); todd.hankinson@childrenscolorado.org (T.H.)
2. Department of Pediatric Neurosurgery, Children's Hospital Colorado, University of Colorado, Aurora, CO 80045, USA
3. Morgan Adams Foundation Pediatric Brain Tumor Program, Aurora, CO 80045, USA
4. Department of Neuropathology, University of Colorado Hospital, Aurora, CO 80045, USA; Ahmed.Gilani@childrenscolorado.org
* Correspondence: ros.whelan@cuamschutz.edu

Received: 2 January 2020; Accepted: 12 February 2020; Published: 14 February 2020

Abstract: Pediatric Adamantinomatous Craniopharyngiomas (ACPs) are histologically benign brain tumors that often follow an aggressive clinical course. Their suprasellar location leaves them in close proximity to critical neurological and vascular structures and often results in significant neuroendocrine morbidity. Current treatment paradigms, involving surgical resection and radiotherapy, confer significant morbidity to patients and there is an obvious need to discover effective and safe alternative treatments. Recent years have witnessed significant efforts to fully detail the genomic, transcriptomic and proteomic make-up of these tumors, in an attempt to identify potential therapeutic targets. These studies have resulted in ever mounting evidence that inflammatory processes and the immune response play a critical role in the pathogenesis of both the solid and cystic portion of ACPs. Several inflammatory and immune markers have been identified in both the cyst fluid and solid tumor tissue of ACP. Due to the existence of effective agents that target them, IL-6 and immune checkpoint inhibitors seem to present the most likely immediate candidates for clinical trials of targeted immune-related therapy in ACP. If effective, such agents may result in a paradigm shift in treatment that ultimately reduces morbidity and results in better outcomes for our patients.

Keywords: craniopharyngioma; inflammation; checkpoint inhibitors; Interleukin-6

1. Introduction

Pediatric Adamantinomatous Craniopharyngiomas (ACPs) are histologically benign brain tumors that often follow an aggressive clinical course. The tumors are most commonly centered in the suprasellar region and are believed to develop from remnants of Rathke's pouch. Radiologically and grossly, these tumors appear as mixed solid and cystic lesions often with areas of calcification (Figure 1). Histologically, ACPs are heterogeneous tumors of epithelial origin [1,2]. The classic features consist of palisading epithelium, stellate cells, nodules of anuclear "ghost cells" and "wet keratin" as well as large areas of regressive changes (i.e., inflammation and calcifications, multinucleated giant cells, hemosiderin deposits, cholesterol clefts) [1] (Figure 2). Their proximity to critical neurological and vascular structures often confers significant neuroendocrine morbidity on patients [3]. Surgery remains the primary treatment strategy, but can result in significant morbidity, specifically damage to the hypothalamus, pituitary and optic apparatus, which results in long-term sequelae that can greatly impact a child's quality of life [4–6]. In an era of personalized medicine and targeted therapies,

ACP remains resistant to such advances. On the other hand, recent case reports of the response of papillary craniopharyngioma, a different tumor of the suprasellar region, to BRAF inhibitors have elucidated the great potential of targeted therapies in treating these tumors [7,8]. As a result, recent years have witnessed significant efforts to fully elucidate the genomic, transcriptomic and proteomic make-up of ACP in an attempt to identify potential therapeutic targets for the treatment of this disease [9–15].

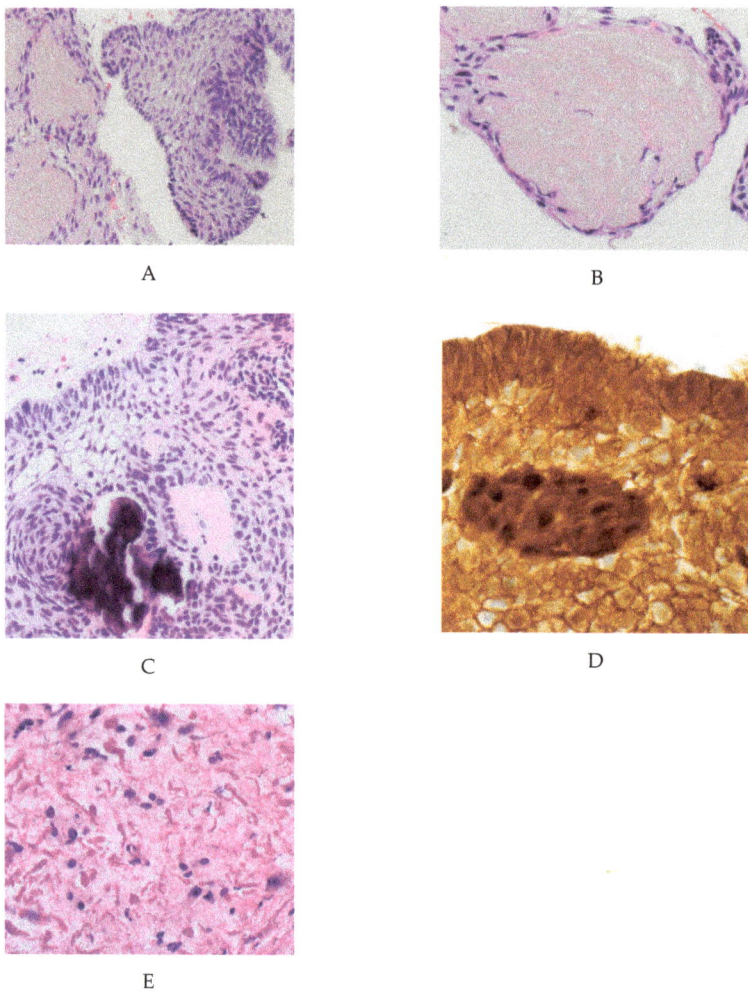

Figure 1. Classic histopathological findings in adamantinomatous craniopharyngioma: (**A**) H&E stained sections showing an epithelial tumor with palisading cells with aggregates of 'wet' keratin; (**B**) higher magnification view demonstrating keratinized 'ghost cells'; (**C**) Higher magnification view demonstrating calcifications and stellate reticulum; (**D**) Immunohistochemical staining for Beta-catenin that is nuclear positive in a subset of tumor cells. (**E**) The surrounding brain parenchyma shows extensive gliosis with Rosenthal fibers.

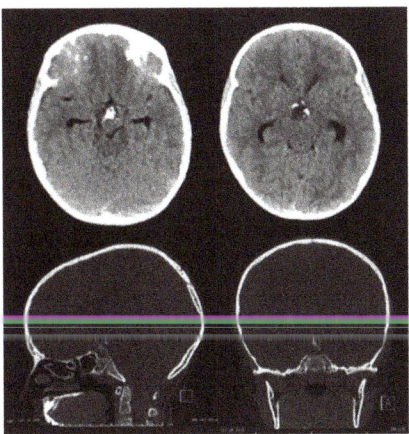 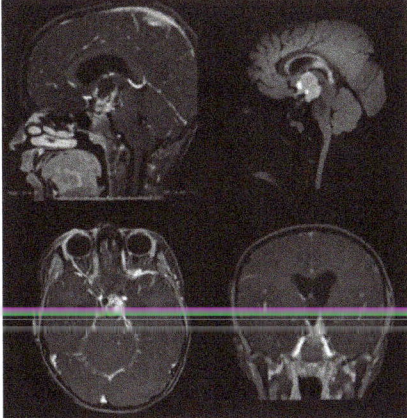

Figure 2. Computed Tomography (**Left**) and Magnetic resonance Imaging (**Right**) images from the same patient of a classic example of an adamantinomatous craniopharyngioma. This typical tumor is centered in the suprasellar region with mixed solid and cystic areas as well as areas of calcification as seen on the CT.

1.1. The Central Role of WNT Pathway Overactivation in the Tumorigenesis of ACP

The one consistent genomic mutation that appears to be present in the majority, if not all, of ACPs is an activation mutation in the *CTNNB1* gene of the WNT/wingless pathway [9,11,16]. Most commonly this involves a point mutation in exon 3 of the *CTNNB1* gene. A number of studies have demonstrated various different mutations, most commonly involving serine or threonine phosphorylation sites encoded by exon 3 [13,17]. Ordinarily, and in the absence of WNT activation, beta-catenin is marked for destruction by a destruction complex consisting of AXIN, glycogen synthase kinase-3β (GSK3β), and APC, among other proteins. This complex binds to and phosphorylates specific residues encoded by exon 3 of *CTNNB1* and results in degradation of the protein [13,18]. In the presence of WNT activation, WNT ligands bind to Frizzled and its co-receptor LRP (Low-density lipoprotein receptor-related protein) at the cell membrane. This in turn leads to the activation of Disheveled (DVL) and the binding of AXIN at the cell membrane. Consequently, the normal destruction complex is broken up and beta-catenin is released. Eventually this stabilized beta-catenin will accumulate in first the cytoplasm, and subsequently the nucleus resulting in the expression of WNT pathway target genes [18]. In the pathological state present in ACP, the various point mutations prevent the binding of GSK3β to beta-catenin, and the subsequent phosphorylation of the serine and threonine residues. This results in a degradation-resistant form of beta-catenin, resulting in aberrant nuclear accumulation of the protein in certain cells within the tumor. In the nucleus, beta-catenin acts as a transcription factor, leading to overactivation of the WNT/beta-catenin pathway [16,18,19]. Although this aberrant overactivation of the WNT pathway is thought to be crucial in the pathogenesis of ACPs, the resulting nuclear accumulation of beta-catenin is only observed in a minority of cells, specifically in whorl like epithelial cell clusters (Figure 1D). These cells are thought to be crucial in the tumorigenesis of ACP and various mechanisms have been proposed as to how they may drive tumor growth [16,20,21] (Figure 2).

One such theory involves a paracrine mechanism whereby these cell clusters induce tumor growth by expressing a large array of growth factors, chemokines, and cytokines and act as a kind of signaling center that promotes tumor progression [21]. It has also been hypothesized that the nuclear accumulation of beta-catenin and overactivation of the WNT pathway in these cell clusters might also play a crucial role in the invasion of adjacent structures (e.g. hypothalamus and pituitary) in ACP [20]. Microscopically, a digitate invasion/growth pattern into structures such as the hypothalamus can be seen and is thought to be an important factor in the neuro-endocrine disorders frequently seen in children with ACP [3,22]. In addition, this invasive nature can preclude the neurosurgeon from obtaining a gross total resection at the time of surgery leading to tumor recurrence and a more aggressive clinical course. Hölsken et al. [20] noted that beta-catenin accumulating whorls/clusters are found at the tips of these invading projections of tumor and hypothesized that this may suggest a role for these clusters in the promotion of tumor invasion [20]. In addition, Apps et al. [23] used micro-CT to produce 3-D models of ACP tumor samples. Using this novel technique, they visualized cell clusters in tumor protrusions into surrounding tissue. In a separate paper, the same group used laser capture microdissection to separate out these cell clusters and analyze their transcriptomic profiles [10]. They found that these cell clusters express high levels of the FGF, BMP and WNT families of secreted factors and were able to demonstrate downstream activation of the MAPK/ERK that was particularly prominent at the tips of the invading tumor epithelium. These facts lend further credence to the theory that these clusters drive tumor invasion in a paracrine manner. Hölsken et al. [20] cultured a total of 6 ACP samples and measured their invasion capacity via two methods, namely Boyden chamber assays, and wound-healing assays. They then suppressed beta-catenin expression in the samples by introducing small interfering RNA (siRNA) directed against the *CTNNB1* gene and repeated the assays. They found that after treatment with the siRNA the accumulation of beta-catenin was significantly reduced and resulted in a significant decrease in tumor cell migration and invasion capacity [20]. They also demonstrated that the treatment with siRNA resulted in the reduced expression of the Fascin protein. Fascin is a member of the actin cross-linking family of proteins and plays a crucial role in cell-matrix adhesion, cell migration, and remodeling of the cell cytoskeleton/architecture [24,25]. In addition, the aberrant overexpression of the Fascin protein has been demonstrated in a number of cancers, including oral squamous cell carcinoma, and prostate cancer [24,26]. Hölsken et al. [20] demonstrated that the beta-catenin accumulating cells in ACP also over expressed Fascin. They then showed that treatment with the siRNA lead to a decrease in not only beta-catenin accumulation, but also Fascin levels. They proposed that this increase in Fascin expression may represent the mechanism by which WNT overactivation in these ACP cells may increase tumor cell migration and invasion into adjacent structures [20].

Given the seemingly crucial role of WNT overactivation in ACPs, targeting the WNT pathway would appear to represent an attractive strategy for tackling these tumors. The WNT pathway has been shown to play a crucial role in a number of cancers such as colorectal cancers, non-small cell lung cancer, and chronic myeloid leukemia [27,28]. This has resulted in significant efforts to better understand the pathway and to develop therapies that target it [27,28]. Despite all these efforts, no drug targeting the WNT pathway has been approved. The reasons for the difficulty in targeting the WNT pathway are legion and complex but one major area of concern is the important role the pathway plays in the maintenance of normal stem cells for tissue regeneration [27,29]. The potential issues that may arise with WNT pathway targeting was illustrated by Zhong et al. [30] who demonstrated significant intestinal toxicity associated with tankyrase inhibitors in mice.

Due to the difficulties that have been encountered in targeting the WNT pathway in more aggressive cancers, it seems likely that such therapies with acceptable efficacy and toxicity will remain elusive for some time to come [28]. It is unlikely such a therapy will become a viable option in the treatment of ACP in the near future and as a result, the need to discover other effective therapies has become imperative. ACP is a very rare disease and developing novel therapies specifically for this tumor type is currently not practical or realistic. As a result, much work has focused on identifying alternative targets with extant treatments, which may offer better results in the treatment of ACP. These efforts have resulted in the identification of multiple molecular pathways involved in the pathogenesis of ACP [6]. A number of these pathways result in the upregulation of pro-inflammatory/immune genes that may be amenable to targeted therapies [10,11,31–33]. The immune/inflammatory cells seen in ACP samples are varied and can include CD4-T-Lymphocytes, CD20-B-Lymphocytes, CD-68-Macrophages, and CD-56-NK cells. The presence of all these cells is not consistent among all ACP samples and this fact is reflective of the histologically heterogeneous nature of these tumors [34]. Work is ongoing to investigate whether these pathways may present potential therapeutic targets and ultimately leads to better outcomes and reduced morbidity for patients. The following is a review of the evidence that highlights the potential importance of the inflammatory/immune response in the generation of these tumors and the potential in targeting these pathways in the treatment of this often-devastating disease.

1.2. The role of the Inflammatory Response in Generating the Cystic Compartment in ACP

ACPs often have large cystic components that contribute to the adverse clinical outcomes associated with the disease (Figure 3). Their large size and at times rapid growth can injure or exert mass effect on critical adjacent structures, such as the pituitary, the hypothalamus, the optic apparatus and third ventricle, which may necessitate urgent surgical intervention to preserve function and prevent morbidity and mortality. As a result, a better understanding of the pathogenesis of ACP cysts and the development of better treatments to limit their growth is clearly desirable. Numerous studies have analyzed the content of these cysts and the results of these studies have demonstrated a significant inflammatory content within them. A summary of some of these papers is presented in Table 1.

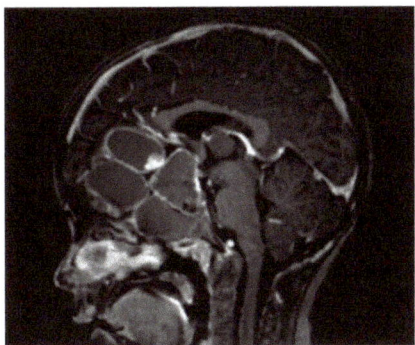

Figure 3. Example of an adamantinomatous craniopharyngioma with a massive cystic component.

Table 1. Key studies that have demonstrated the key role of the inflammatory/immune response in the pathogenesis of adamantinomatous craniopharyngioma.

Study	Summary of Study	Findings
Kilday et al. 2017 [35]	Multinational study assessing the efficacy of intra-cystic IFN-alpha in treating ACP	Demonstrated a progression free survival advantage for intracystic IFN-alpha
Pettorini et al. 2010 [36]	Identified the presence of alpha-defensins 1–3 in ACP cyst fluid	Demonstrated the importance of inflammation the genesis of ACP cysts
Gump et al. 2015 [11]	Used mRNA microarray analysis to identify the overexpression of multiple inflammatory markers in ACP relative to other tumors	Identifies IL6R and IL2RB to be overexpressed in ACP relative to normal brain and other tumors
Donson et al. 2017 [31]	Identified elevated levels of severeal inflammatory markers in both ACP cyst fluid and solid tumor	Overexpressed inflammatory markers identified included IL-6, IL-8, CXCL1, and IL-10
Apps et al. 2018 [10]	Used various methods including RNA sequencing to identify activation of the inflammasome in ACP cyst fluid and solid tumor	Imflatory genes that were overexpressed included IL-1B, IL-18, IL-6, IL-8, IL-10
Coy et al. 2018 [33]	demonstrated the expression of PD-L1 in epithelial cells lining the cysts and intrinsic PD-1 expression in the beta-catenin over expressing whorl-like epithelial cell clusters in ACP	The first paper to demonstrate that immune checkpoint inhibitors may play a role in ACP treatments

Some of the first work examining the role of inflammation in ACP pathogenesis was carried out by Mori et al. who demonstrated highly elevated levels of IL-6 in the cyst fluid of 15 pediatric ACPs and posited that IL-6 plays an important role in the inflammatory reaction associated with ACPs [37]. Another study that demonstrated the role played by the inflammatory response in the generation of the ACP cyst was that by Pettorini et al. [36]. Using high-performance liquid chromatography and mass spectrometry to analyze cyst fluid from 6 patients, they found high levels of alpha defensins 1–3, proteins that are present in neutrophils and are involved in the inflammatory-mediated response. Furthermore, their group demonstrated that these levels were significantly reduced after treatment with intracystic interferon alpha (IFN-alpha). They posited that the detection of these proteins suggested that the innate immune response was playing a critical role in cyst generation and that a possible mechanism of action of IFN-alpha in treating the cyst was via an immune-modulatory effect [36]. A later study by the same group performed more extensive proteomic analysis on nineteen patient samples [15]. In this study, they used reverse phase liquid chromatography in conjunction with high resolution ESI-I TQ-Orbitrap mass spectrometry to analyze ACP cyst fluid from nineteen children. In addition to again revealing elevated levels of alpha-defensins (that again were reduced after treatment with IFN-alpha), they also demonstrated elevated levels of several other proteins of inflammation. Specifically, these included alpha2-HS-glycoprotein, alpha1-antichymotrypsin and apolipoproteins.

In another study, Donson et al. [31] used cytometric bead analysis to measure the concentration of 24 cytokines and 11 chemokines in cyst fluid from five pediatric ACPs and five pediatric pilocytic astrocytomas (PAs). Their analysis demonstrated that six cytokines were present at statistically significant increased levels in ACPs versus PAs. These cytokines included IL-6, IL-10, CXCL8 (IL-8), and CXCL1 (GRO). Of these, levels of IL-6 demonstrated the greatest difference between ACPs and PAs. Apps et al. also demonstrated similar findings when analyzing the protein content of ACP cyst fluid [10]. They analyzed the content of cyst fluid from 6 patients with ACP using multiplex ELISA (Enzyme-linked immunosorbent assay). They found that the cyst fluid contained several proteins associated with inflammation, such as apolipoproteins, complement system proteins and immunoglobulins. In addition, their analysis revealed the presence of cytokines such as IL-1B, IL-6, IL-8, IL-10, IL-18 as well as TNF (Tumor necrosis factor) and Interferon gamma.

Further evidence for the role of inflammation in the genesis of the cystic component in ACPs is provided by the efficacy of treatment with IFN-alpha. IFN-alpha has been used with varying degrees of success in the treatment of multiple cancers [38]. The mechanism of action in the treatment of neoplasms is complex and multifaceted but likely involves the stimulation of an anti-cancer immune response [38]. The use of intracystic IFN-alpha in the treatment of cystic ACP has been established for several years and numerous studies have demonstrated its safety and efficacy [35,39,40]. The treatment involves the surgical placement of a catheter within the cyst with the position of the catheter confirmed radiologically prior to the administration of the drug. This method of treatment has been shown to delay disease progression and can allow the clinical team to delay a more definitive treatment via surgical resection and radiotherapy [35]. Such a delay is often desirable, as it by may allow a child's developing brain to mature further prior to undergoing inherently risky surgery and radiation therapy. The mechanism of action of intracystic IFN-alpha in treating ACP has not been confirmed but, as in other cancers, is likely to involve an immunomodulatory effect. Indeed, the previously mentioned proteomic analyses would seem to lend significant weight to this argument [36].

1.3. The Solid Component of ACP Also Demonstrates Elevated Levels of Several Inflammatory Markers

Multiple studies have also identified high levels of cytokines and inflammatory markers in the solid component of ACPs, lending further support to the theory that inflammation plays a critical role in pathogenesis [18,31]. Gump et al. used micro-array data to demonstrate elevated levels of IL-6R in ACP relative to other pediatric brain tumors [11]. Subsequently, Donson et al. [31], utilized detailed transcriptomic analysis to demonstrate increased expression of pro-inflammatory mediators in ACP solid tumor tissue including IL-6, CXCL1, CLCL8, CXCR2, IL-10 and IDO-1. Separate work by Martelli et al. [32] used advanced proteomics to investigate the protein signature in ACP. In addition to identifying beta-catenin and its related proteins in solid tumor tissue from seven patients, their analysis also identified the presence of increased levels of alpha-defensins 1–4. As previously stated, these proteins are neutrophil-derived proteins that play an important role in the innate immune response and in inflammation. Their detection in the solid portion of ACP again seems to confirm that the inflammatory response plays an important role in ACP tumorigenesis.

A recent paper by Apps et al. used transcriptome analysis of tumor tissue from 18 patients to identify a pattern of elevated expression of several immune cell markers and immune system genes in ACP [10]. Furthermore, their analysis used immunohistochemistry to reveal the presence of both myeloid-derived and lymphoid-derived cells infiltrating both the reactive glial and tumor epithelial compartments in the ACP samples. They also found that multiple cytokine encoding genes were highly upregulated in ACP and that the expression of such genes correlated with the immune infiltrate and inflammatory cell markers. This would suggest that this upregulated cytokine expression is mostly derived from the infiltrating immune cells rather than from the tumor cells that are over expressing beta-catenin. Finally, they also utilized multiplex ELISA to analyze protein lysates from eight patient ACP samples and this analysis revealed the expression of IL-1B, Il-6, IL-8, IL-10, IL-18, and TNF-alpha in all the samples.

1.4. Immune Checkpoint Inhibitors and Their Potential Use in ACP

Immune checkpoint inhibitors have shown promise in the treatment of a number of cancers. Specifically, inhibition of the programmed cell death protein (PD1) and its ligand (PD-L1) with the agents, nivolumab and pembrolizumab, has resulted in improved survival in cancers including melanoma and non-small cell lung adenocarcinoma [41,42]. The availability of these agents and their relatively favorable side effect profile has resulted in numerous studies investigating their efficacy in various cancers/tumor types.

PD-1 is an important protein involved in inhibitory immune signaling and is an essential regulator of the adaptive immune response [43]. In cancers, PD-1-expressing tumor-infiltrating T cells can be disabled by PD-L1 expressed on the surfaces of tumor cells themselves or alternatively by PD-L1 on the surface of other infiltrating immune cells. The binding of PD-1 to its ligand results in the suppression of the immune response to the cancer cells [43,44]. Checkpoint Inhibitors reverse this process and allow T cells to once again attack the cancer. Predicting the response of a particular tumor or cancer to PD1 inhibitors such as nivolumab and pembrolizumab is difficult and Taube et al. aimed to identify those factors that best predicted a robust and meaningful response to therapy [44]. In a prior study by the same group they found that anti-PD-1 therapy produced an objective response in 20–25% of patients with treatment-resistant NSCLC, renal cell carcinoma and melanoma and that PD-L1 expression by tumor cells seemed to be associated with a response to therapy [45]. In their follow up study they aimed to further investigate various factors that might predict a response to anti-PD-1 therapy including PD-L1 expression by tumor cells, PD-L1 expression by infiltrating immune cells, PD-L2 expression by tumor cells and other tumor microenvironment factors. They found that in their cohort only the expression of PD-L1 by tumor cells correlated with both an objective response (as defined by the "Response evaluation criteria in Solid Tumors" or RECIST criteria) and clinical benefit ($p = 0.025$ and 0.005 respectively). The correlation of the expression of PD-L1 by infiltrating immune cells with a clinical response did not reach statistical significance although the correlation with clinical benefit was statistically significant ($p = 0.038$). Of note, expression of the PD-1 receptor on tumor infiltrating lymphocytes (TILs), expression of PD-L2 by tumor cells or TILs, and other microenvironment immune factors did not correlate with outcomes. In addition, it is important to reiterate that even in those tumors expressing PD-L1 on tumor cells, only 39% of patients (9 out of 23) had an objective response [44]. That being said, these therapies have provided an option for patients with aggressive and treatment-resistant cancers for whom previously there were few if any good options. Due to the efficacy of immune checkpoint inhibitors more and more work is being undertaken to identify other cancers and tumors that may be amenable to such therapy including craniopharyngiomas.

Recent work by Coy et al. [33] demonstrated the expression of PD-L1 in epithelial cells lining the cysts and intrinsic PD-1 expression in the beta-catenin over expressing whorl-like epithelial cell clusters in ACP. As previously discussed, these clusters are thought to play a pivotal role in tumor growth in ACP via a number of mechanisms [13,20,21], rendering targeting of PD-1 as an attractive potential therapy. Another study by Witt et al. [46] also demonstrated elevated PD-L1 expression in ACP. As mentioned above, numerous previous studies on other solid cancers have demonstrated that the expression of PD-L1 can be predictive of the response to the PD-1/PD-L1 inhibitors [44,45]. Again, as previously mentioned, such a finding far from guarantees a response and in these landmark papers they found that even in patients that expressed PD-L1 on tumor cells, the response rate to the treatment was only 39% [44]. In addition, Witt et al. [46] nicely demonstrated, using T cell exhaustion testing of various types of ependymomas, that elevated PD-L1 expression in tumors can be indicative of either tumor adaptations to hide from the innate immune response or due to normal T-cell antigen-activation, a known function of PD-1. In their study they utilized functional T cell exhaustion assays that stimulate T cells via exposure to Phorbol 12-myristate 13-acetate (PMA)/ionomycin. Subsequent to stimulations their group used a Milliplex Map Kit (Millipore) to measure the concentration of several cytokines including IFN-gamma. They found that infiltrating T-cells in RELA fusion supratentorial ependymoma did not secrete IFN-gamma. They concluded that this suggested that in the case of RELA fusion ependymoma, the increased expression of PD-1/PD-L1 results in the exhaustion of infiltrating T-cells and immune evasion by the tumor [46]. On the contrary, they found that in group B ependymomas (which also express high levels of PD-1), infiltrating T-cells were, in fact, capable of secreting IFN-gamma after stimulation with PMA/ionomycin. They posited that in these tumors, elevated expression of PD-1 was representative of normal T-cell activation in response to the tumor [46]. As such, although the findings by Coy et al. [33] of elevated PD-1/PD-L1 expression in ACP are exciting and may result in an alternative treatment strategy in resistant and multiply recurrent cases, further investigation is necessary to fully elucidate the implications of this increased PD-1/PD-L1 expression in ACP before any widespread implementation.

1.5. CTLA-4 Inhibition and Its Potential Use in the Treatment of ACP

The other major group of immune checkpoint inhibitors that have become increasingly utilized in cancer are the CTLA-4 inhibitors of which ipilimumab is the classic example. One of the first major studies to demonstrate the efficacy of these agents was that by Hodi et al. [47] in 2010. In their study they randomized 676 patients with stage 3 or 4 treatment-resistant melanoma to treatment with ipilimumab plus glycoprotein 100 (gp100) or gp100 alone. They demonstrated a statistically significant, although modest benefit, in terms of survival for patients in the ipilimumab group. Subsequent work by Ji et al. aimed to elucidate what specific factors might be predictive of response to treatment with CTLA-4 blockade [48]. This group utilized gene expression profiling to demonstrate that in pre-treatment samples of patients with metastatic melanoma a higher baseline expression of immune related genes was predictive of an increased response to treatment with ipilimumab [48]. Specifically, they analyzed the gene expression in tumor samples from 45 patients with melanoma both before, and three weeks after treatment with ipilimumab. They found that tumors that had increased expression of immune related genes pre-treatment, were more likely to respond to the therapy. Indeed, when they clustered genes based on biological functions and examined the differential expression of these groups of genes between responders and non-responders, they demonstrated that genes related to the inflammatory response were those that were most differentially expressed between the two groups [48]. This led their group to conclude that a "pre-existing immune-active tumor microenvironment might favor clinical response to ipilimumab". As previously stated, ACPs have been shown to harbor a significant inflammatory/immune component in both the solid and cystic component and there is mounting evidence that this pro-inflammatory environment plays an active role in tumorigenesis [31]. A 2017 study by Donson et al. [31] utilized various methods to demonstrate upregulation of several pro-inflammatory genes in both the solid and cystic component of these tumors. This begs the question, could the use of a CTLA-4 inhibitor such as ipilimumab lead to improved outcomes in ACP? Furthermore, recent trials have demonstrated that combining different types of immune checkpoint inhibitors can lead to a survival advantage for patients with treatment refractory cancers. Specifically, combining ant-PD1 and anti-CTLA-4 therapy can result in improved survival in treatment-resistant metastatic melanoma, renal cell carcinoma and non-small cell lung cancer [49–52]. Given the expression of PD-L1 and the significant immune cell and inflammatory milieu present in ACP, the use of such combinations in the treatment of this disease would appear promising. As a result, a lot of work remains to be done to fully elucidate the potential of such treatments in ACP. Given the often-aggressive clinical course, and devastating effects this disease can have on patient's quality of life such potential is surely worth investigating.

1.6. The Role of Senescence and the Senescence Associated Secretory Phenotype (SASP) in the Pathogenesis of ACP

In the normal physiological state, cellular senescence develops in response to both extracellular and intracellular stressors and pushes the cell into cell cycle arrest. This prevents propagation of the damaged cell and, when this occurs in the context of cancer, can ultimately result in tumor suppression [53]. Paradoxically, senescent cells can go on to develop secretory functions that result in changes to the cellular microenvironment and may ultimately promote tumor growth [53]. Senescent cells can persist in a metabolically active state, ultimately developing what is termed the Senescence Associated Secretory Phenotype (SASP) [53]. In such a state, cells can secrete a variety of interleukins, inflammatory cytokines, growth factors, and proteases, which can affect the surrounding cells and tumor microenvironment. SASP factors include pro-inflammatory mediators such as IL-6, IL-1, certain Matrix Metalloproteinases, and various chemokines [53,54]. Of these, Rodier et al. [54] found that IL-6 was the most important in allowing senescent cells to promote cell invasion. Gonzalez-Meljem et al. [55] demonstrated that the SASP plays a prominent role in both genetically engineered mouse models of ACP and human ACP. They used gene set enrichment analysis (GSEA) to demonstrate that beta-catenin accumulating cluster cells in the mouse models of ACP had gene expression profiles that were significantly enriched for SASP genes. Similarly, they utilized ELISA cytokine arrays to demonstrate that multiple SASP associated proteins such as IL-6, IL-1a, MMP2, MMP3, CXCL1, and CXCL11 were all upregulated in the murine cluster cells [55]. In addition, other studies, such as those by Gump et al. [11], and Apps et al. [10], used various techniques to demonstrate the overexpression of several of these proteins in human ACP. Meljem et al. [55] then used laser-capture microdissection and RNA sequencing to analyze the molecular signature of the beta-catenin accumulating cell clusters in human ACP. They performed hierarchical clustering analysis that demonstrated similar molecular profiles between the cluster cells from the mouse models and those from human ACP. Subsequent GSEA of human clusters also demonstrated a strong SASP signature. They thus concluded that the human and mouse clusters represent equivalent structures and share a common senescent molecular signature. Given the critical role that these cell clusters are thought to play in ACP tumorigenesis, they posited that the SASP may play a critical role in the pathogenesis of ACP [55]. This paper aimed to demonstrate the critical role played by inflammation in the pathogenesis of ACP. Given that human ACPs seem to harbor a very strong SASP signature and the SASP induces a strong pro-inflammatory state, it is very possible that the SASP plays a critical role in producing the pro-inflammatory milieu and invasive nature of ACP. Trials examining the use of senolytic drugs are currently in their incipient stages and it is possible that such therapies may provide an attractive treatment strategy for ACP in the future [56].

2. Conclusions

A significant and growing body of evidence points to a critical role in the activation of inflammation and the immune response in the pathogenesis of ACP. Multiple studies have demonstrated high levels of inflammatory markers and cytokines in both ACP cyst fluid and solid tumor. Many of these employed advanced genomic, proteomic and transcriptomic techniques to demonstrate expression of multiple genes involved in the inflammatory and immune response in these tumors. A number of these markers represent attractive potential targets for directed therapy in the treatment of ACP. Specifically, due to existing experience combined with proven efficacy in other cancers and diseases, IL-6 and the immune checkpoint inhibitors (anti-PD-1/PD-L1 and anti-CTLA-4) may represent particularly good targets/therapies. Similarly, combinations of such agents have proven very effective in prolonging survival in malignant cancer such as melanoma, renal cell carcinoma and non-small-cell lung cancer that were failing more traditional treatment. Such combination therapy may also present a potential therapeutic strategy in the management of recurrent and treatment-resistant ACP. In addition, these agents might also be combined with agents that do not specifically interact with inflammatory/immune processes (e.g., MEK inhibition). In fact, Apps et al. [10] demonstrated that MAPK/ERK pathway likely plays a pivotal role in the pathogenesis of both murine and human ACP. In addition, they showed that treating human ACP with trametinib ex vivo resulted in decreased proliferation and increased apoptosis. Finally, recent work has also demonstrated the pivotal role played by senescence and the SASP in the pathogenesis of these tumors. It is possible that the strong SASP signature drives much of the inflammation seen in ACP, and that targeting SASP associated pathways may provide an effective treatment strategy in the future. Due to the benign histological nature of the disease, it is likely that initial clinical trials of such agents will be reserved for patients with recurrent or progressive disease. In addition, due to the rarity of the disease and the scarcity of tumor tissue it is vital that pediatric centers continue to work together to share knowledge and tissue in an effort to accelerate the development of safe and efficacious treatments. Such efforts will hopefully result in improved outcomes for children suffering from this chronic and often devastating disease. Finally, other advanced techniques are being developed that continue to enhance our ability to better diagnose, and identify biomarkers in oncologic diseases that may result in the development of better therapeutics [57,58]. It is possible that such techniques if applied to ACPs could result in significant advances in the diagnosis and treatment of ACP in the future.

Author Contributions: R.W. as the first author was primarily responsible for drafting the article manuscript. E.P. also helped draft the manuscript and helped with editing the final submission. A.G. provided the pathology figures and the descriptions of the same. T.H. acted as the lead author and guided the direction of the manuscript as well as being the primary editor of the final submission. All authors have read and agreed to the published version of the manuscript.

Funding: No external funding was received for the production of this research.

Conflicts of Interest: The authors declare no conflict of interest.

References

1. Martinez-Barbera, J.P.; Buslei, R. Adamantinomatous craniopharyngioma: Pathology, molecular genetics and mouse models. *J. Pediatr. Endocrinol. Metab.* **2015**, *28*, 7–17. [CrossRef]
2. Kasai, H.; Hirano, A.; Llena, J.F.; Kawamoto, K. A histopathological study of craniopharyngioma with special reference to its stroma and surrounding tissue. *Brain Tumor Pathol.* **1997**, *14*, 41–45. [CrossRef] [PubMed]
3. Daubenbüchel, A.; Müller, H. Neuroendocrine Disorders in Pediatric Craniopharyngioma Patients. *J. Clin. Med.* **2015**, *4*, 389–413. [CrossRef] [PubMed]
4. Müller, H.L.; Gebhardt, U.; Teske, C.; Faldum, A.; Zwiener, I.; Warmuth-Metz, M.; Pietsch, T.; Pohl, F.; Sörensen, N.; Calaminus, G. Post-operative hypothalamic lesions and obesity in childhood craniopharyngioma: Results of the multinational prospective trial KRANIOPHARYNGEOM 2000 after 3-year follow-up. *Eur. J. Endocrinol.* **2011**, *165*, 17–24. [CrossRef] [PubMed]

5. Heinks, K.; Boekhoff, S.; Hoffmann, A.; Warmuth-Metz, M.; Eveslage, M.; Peng, J.; Calaminus, G.; Müller, H.L. Quality of life and growth after childhood craniopharyngioma: Results of the multinational trial KRANIOPHARYNGEOM 2007. *Endocrine* **2018**, *59*, 364–372. [CrossRef]
6. Müller, H.L.; Merchant, T.E.; Puget, S.; Martinez-Barbera, J.P. New outlook on the diagnosis, treatment and follow-up of childhood-onset craniopharyngioma. *Nat. Rev. Endocrinol.* **2017**, *13*, 299–312. [CrossRef]
7. Brastianos, P.K.; Shankar, G.M.; Gill, C.M.; Taylor-Weiner, A.; Nayyar, N.; Panka, D.J.; Sullivan, R.J.; Frederick, D.T.; Abedalthagafi, M.; Jones, P.S.; et al. Dramatic Response of BRAF V600E Mutant Papillary Craniopharyngioma to Targeted Therapy. *J. Natl. Cancer Inst.* **2015**, *108*. [CrossRef]
8. Aylwin, S.J.B.; Bodi, I.; Beaney, R. Pronounced response of papillary craniopharyngioma to treatment with vemurafenib, a BRAF inhibitor. *Pituitary* **2016**, *19*, 544–546. [CrossRef]
9. Brastianos, P.K.; Taylor-Weiner, A.; Manley, P.E.; Jones, R.T.; Dias-Santagata, D.; Thorner, A.R.; Lawrence, M.S.; Rodriguez, F.J.; Bernardo, L.A.; Schubert, L.; et al. Exome sequencing identifies BRAF mutations in papillary craniopharyngiomas. *Nat. Genet.* **2014**, *46*, 161–165. [CrossRef]
10. Apps, J.R.; Carreno, G.; Gonzalez-Meljem, J.M.; Haston, S.; Guiho, R.; Cooper, J.E.; Manshaei, S.; Jani, N.; Hölsken, A.; Pettorini, B.; et al. Tumour compartment transcriptomics demonstrates the activation of inflammatory and odontogenic programmes in human adamantinomatous craniopharyngioma and identifies the MAPK/ERK pathway as a novel therapeutic target. *Acta Neuropathol.* **2018**, *135*, 757–777. [CrossRef] [PubMed]
11. Gump, J.M.; Donson, A.M.; Birks, D.K.; Amani, V.M.; Rao, K.K.; Griesinger, A.M.; Kleinschmidt-DeMasters, B.K.; Johnston, J.M.; Anderson, R.C.E.; Rosenfeld, A.; et al. Identification of targets for rational pharmacological therapy in childhood craniopharyngioma. *Acta Neuropathol. Commun.* **2015**, *3*, 30. [CrossRef]
12. Hölsken, A.; Sill, M.; Merkle, J.; Schweizer, L.; Buchfelder, M.; Flitsch, J.; Fahlbusch, R.; Metzler, M.; Kool, M.; Pfister, S.M.; et al. Adamantinomatous and papillary craniopharyngiomas are characterized by distinct epigenomic as well as mutational and transcriptomic profiles. *Acta Neuropathol. Commun.* **2016**, *4*, 20. [CrossRef]
13. Goschzik, T.; Gessi, M.; Dreschmann, V.; Gebhardt, U.; Wang, L.; Yamaguchi, S.; Wheeler, D.A.; Lauriola, L.; Lau, C.C.; Müller, H.L.; et al. Genomic Alterations of Adamantinomatous and Papillary Craniopharyngioma. *J. Neuropathol. Exp. Neurol.* **2017**, *76*, 126–134. [CrossRef]
14. Andoniadou, C.L.; Gaston-Massuet, C.; Reddy, R.; Schneider, R.P.; Blasco, M.A.; Le Tissier, P.; Jacques, T.S.; Pevny, L.H.; Dattani, M.T.; Martinez-Barbera, J.P. Identification of novel pathways involved in the pathogenesis of human adamantinomatous craniopharyngioma. *Acta Neuropathol.* **2012**, *124*, 259–271. [CrossRef]
15. Massimi, L.; Martelli, C.; Caldarelli, M.; Castagnola, M.; Desiderio, C. Proteomics in pediatric cystic craniopharyngioma. *Brain Pathol.* **2017**, *27*, 370–376. [CrossRef]
16. Robinson, L.C.; Santagata, S.; Hankinson, T.C. Potential evolution of neurosurgical treatment paradigms for craniopharyngioma based on genomic and transcriptomic characteristics. *Neurosurg. Focus* **2016**, *41*, E3. [CrossRef]
17. Buslei, R.; Nolde, M.; Hofmann, B.; Meissner, S.; Eyupoglu, I.Y.; Siebzehnrübl, F.; Hahnen, E.; Kreutzer, J.; Fahlbusch, R. Common mutations of β-catenin in adamantinomatous craniopharyngiomas but not in other tumours originating from the sellar region. *Acta Neuropathol.* **2005**, *109*, 589–597. [CrossRef]
18. Martinez-Barbera, J.P. Molecular and cellular pathogenesis of adamantinomatous craniopharyngioma. *Neuropathol. Appl. Neurobiol.* **2015**, *41*, 721–732. [CrossRef]
19. Apps, J.R.; Martinez-Barbera, J.P. Genetically engineered mouse models of craniopharyngioma: An opportunity for therapy development and understanding of tumor biology. *Brain Pathol.* **2017**, *27*, 364–369. [CrossRef]
20. Hölsken, A.; Buchfelder, M.; Fahlbusch, R.; Blümcke, I.; Buslei, R. Tumour cell migration in adamantinomatous craniopharyngiomas is promoted by activated Wnt-signalling. *Acta Neuropathol.* **2010**, *119*, 631–639. [CrossRef]
21. Martinez-Barbera, J.P.; Andoniadou, C.L. Concise Review: Paracrine Role of Stem Cells in Pituitary Tumors: A Focus on Adamantinomatous Craniopharyngioma. *Stem Cells* **2016**, *34*, 268–276. [CrossRef] [PubMed]
22. Stache, C.; Hölsken, A.; Schlaffer, S.M.; Hess, A.; Metzler, M.; Frey, B.; Fahlbusch, R.; Flitsch, J.; Buchfelder, M.; Buslei, R. Insights into the infiltrative behavior of adamantinomatous craniopharyngioma in a new xenotransplant mouse model. *Brain Pathol.* **2015**, *25*, 1–10. [CrossRef] [PubMed]
23. Apps, J.R.; Hutchinson, J.C.; Arthurs, O.J.; Virasami, A.; Joshi, A.; Zeller-Plumhoff, B.; Moulding, D.; Jacques, T.S.; Sebire, N.J.; Martinez-Barbera, J.P. Imaging Invasion: Micro-CT imaging of adamantinomatous craniopharyngioma highlights cell type specific spatial relationships of tissue invasion. *Acta Neuropathol. Commun.* **2016**, *4*, 57. [CrossRef] [PubMed]

24. Darnel, A.D.; Behmoaram, E.; Vollmer, R.T.; Corcos, J.; Bijian, K.; Sircar, K.; Su, J.; Jiao, J.; Alaoui-Jamali, M.A.; Bismar, T.A. Fascin regulates prostate cancer cell invasion and is associated with metastasis and biochemical failure in prostate cancer. *Clin. Cancer Res.* **2009**, *15*, 1376–1383. [CrossRef]
25. Kureishy, N.; Sapountzi, V.; Prag, S.; Anilkumar, N.; Adams, J.C. Fascins, and their roles in cell structure and function. *BioEssays* **2002**, *24*, 350–361. [CrossRef]
26. Chen, S.F.; Lin, C.Y.; Chang, Y.C.; Li, J.W.; Fu, E.; Chang, F.N.; Lin, Y.L.; Nieh, S. Effects of small interfering RNAs targeting Fascin on gene expression in oral cancer cells. *J. Oral Pathol. Med.* **2009**, *38*, 722–730. [CrossRef]
27. Krishnamurthy, N.; Kurzrock, R. Targeting the Wnt/beta-catenin pathway in cancer: Update on effectors and inhibitors. *Cancer Treat. Rev.* **2018**, *62*, 50–60. [CrossRef]
28. Zhan, T.; Rindtorff, N.; Boutros, M. Wnt signaling in cancer. *Oncogene* **2017**, *36*, 1461–1473. [CrossRef]
29. Staal, F.J.T.; Sen, J.M. The canonical Wnt signaling pathway plays an important role in lymphopoiesis and hematopoiesis. *Eur. J. Immunol.* **2008**, *38*, 1788–1794. [CrossRef]
30. Zhong, Y.; Katavolos, P.; Nguyen, T.; Lau, T.; Boggs, J.; Sambrone, A.; Kan, D.; Merchant, M.; Harstad, E.; Diaz, D.; et al. Tankyrase Inhibition Causes Reversible Intestinal Toxicity in Mice with a Therapeutic Index < 1. *Toxicol. Pathol.* **2016**, *44*, 267–278.
31. Donson, A.M.; Apps, J.; Griesinger, A.M.; Amani, V.; Witt, D.A.; Anderson, R.C.E.; Niazi, T.N.; Grant, G.; Souweidane, M.; Johnston, J.M.; et al. Molecular analyses reveal inflammatory mediators in the solid component and cyst fluid of human adamantinomatous craniopharyngioma. *J. Neuropathol. Exp. Neurol.* **2017**, *76*, 779–788. [CrossRef] [PubMed]
32. Martelli, C.; Serra, R.; Inserra, I.; Rossetti, D.V.; Iavarone, F.; Vincenzoni, F.; Castagnola, M.; Urbani, A.; Tamburrini, G.; Caldarelli, M.; et al. Investigating the Protein Signature of Adamantinomatous Craniopharyngioma Pediatric Brain Tumor Tissue: Towards the Comprehension of Its Aggressive Behavior. *Dis. Markers* **2019**, *2019*. [CrossRef] [PubMed]
33. Coy, S.; Rashid, R.; Lin, J.R.; Du, Z.; Donson, A.M.; Hankinson, T.C.; Foreman, N.K.; Manley, P.E.; Kieran, M.W.; Reardon, D.A.; et al. Multiplexed immunofluorescence reveals potential PD-1/PD-L1 pathway vulnerabilities in craniopharyngioma. *Neuro. Oncol.* **2018**, *20*, 1101–1112. [CrossRef] [PubMed]
34. Martha Lilia, T.S.; Citlaltepelt, S.L.; Ma Elena, H.C.; Carlos, S.G.; Manuel, C.L. Running Head: Craniopharyngioma and Immune Response. *J. Neurol. Neurosci.* **2015**, *06*, 1–10. [CrossRef]
35. Kilday, J.P.; Caldarelli, M.; Massimi, L.; Chen, R.H.H.; Lee, Y.Y.; Liang, M.L.; Parkes, J.; Naiker, T.; Van Veelen, M.L.; Michiels, E.; et al. Intracystic interferon-alpha in pediatric craniopharyngioma patients: An international multicenter assessment on behalf of SIOPE and ISPN. *Neuro. Oncol.* **2017**, *19*, 1398–1407. [CrossRef] [PubMed]
36. Pettorini, B.L.; Inzitari, R.; Massimi, L.; Tamburrini, G.; Caldarelli, M.; Fanali, C.; Cabras, T.; Messana, I.; Castagnola, M.; Di Rocco, C. The role of inflammation in the genesis of the cystic component of craniopharyngiomas. *Child's Nerv. Syst.* **2010**, *26*, 1779–1784. [CrossRef]
37. Mori, M.; Takeshima, H.; Kuratsu, J.I. Expression of interleukin-6 in human craniopharyngiomas: A possible inducer of tumor-associated inflammation. *Int. J. Nol. Med.* **2004**, *14*, 505–509. [CrossRef]
38. Zitvogel, L.; Galluzzi, L.; Kepp, O.; Smyth, M.J.; Kroemer, G. Type I interferons in anticancer immunity. *Nat. Rev. Immunol.* **2015**, *15*, 405–414. [CrossRef]
39. Cavalheiro, S.; Dastoli, P.A.; Silva, N.S.; Toledo, S.; Lederman, H.; da Silva, M.C. Use of interferon alpha in intratumoral chemotherapy for cystic craniopharyngioma. *Child's Nerv. Syst.* **2005**, *21*, 719–724. [CrossRef]
40. Bartels, U.; Laperriere, N.; Bouffet, E.; Drake, J. Intracystic therapies for cystic craniopharyngioma in childhood. *Front. Endocrinol. (Lausanne)* **2012**, *3*, 39. [CrossRef]
41. Garon, E.B.; Rizvi, N.A.; Hui, R.; Leighl, N.; Balmanoukian, A.S.; Eder, J.P.; Patnaik, A.; Aggarwal, C.; Gubens, M.; Horn, L.; et al. Pembrolizumab for the Treatment of Non–Small-Cell Lung Cancer. *N. Engl. J. Med.* **2015**, *372*, 2018–2028. [CrossRef] [PubMed]
42. Robert, C.; Long, G.V.; Brady, B.; Dutriaux, C.; Maio, M.; Mortier, L.; Hassel, J.C.; Rutkowski, P.; McNeil, C.; Kalinka-Warzocha, E.; et al. Nivolumab in previously untreated melanoma without BRAF mutation. *N. Engl. J. Med.* **2015**, *372*, 320–330. [CrossRef]
43. Seidel, J.A.; Otsuka, A.; Kabashima, K. Anti-PD-1 and Anti-CTLA-4 Therapies in Cancer: Mechanisms of Action, Efficacy, and Limitations. *Front. Oncol.* **2018**, *8*, 86. [CrossRef]

44. Taube, J.M.; Klein, A.; Brahmer, J.R.; Xu, H.; Pan, X.; Kim, J.H.; Chen, L.; Pardoll, D.M.; Topalian, S.L.; Anders, R.A. Association of PD-1, PD-1 ligands, and other features of the tumor immune microenvironment with response to anti-PD-1 therapy. *Clin. Cancer Res.* **2014**, *20*, 5064–5074. [CrossRef] [PubMed]
45. Topalian, S.L.; Hodi, F.; Brahmer, J.R.; Gettinger, S.N.; Smith, D.C.; McDermott, D.F.; Powderly, J.D.; Carvajal, R.D.; Sosman, J.A.; Atkins, M.B.; et al. Safety, activity, and immune correlates of anti–PD-1 antibody in cancer. *N. Engl. J. Med.* **2012**, *366*, 2443–2554. [CrossRef] [PubMed]
46. Witt, D.A.; Donson, A.M.; Amani, V.; Moreira, D.C.; Sanford, B.; Hoffman, L.M.; Handler, M.H.; Levy, J.M.M.; Jones, K.L.; Nellan, A.; et al. Specific expression of PD-L1 in RELA-fusion supratentorial ependymoma: Implications for PD-1-targeted therapy. *Pediatr. Blood Cancer* **2018**, *65*, e26960. [CrossRef]
47. Hodi, F.S.; O'Day, S.J.; McDermott, D.F.; Weber, R.W.; Sosman, J.A.; Haanen, J.B.; Gonzalez, R.; Robert, C.; Schadendorf, D.; Hassel, J.C.; et al. Improved survival with ipilimumab in patients with metastatic melanoma. *N. Engl. J. Med.* **2010**, *363*, 711–723. [CrossRef]
48. Ji, R.R.; Chasalow, S.D.; Wang, L.; Hamid, O.; Schmidt, H.; Cogswell, J.; Alaparthy, S.; Berman, D.; Jure-Kunkel, M.; Siemers, N.O.; et al. An immune-active tumor microenvironment favors clinical response to ipilimumab. *Cancer Immunol. Immunother.* **2012**, *61*, 1019–1031. [CrossRef]
49. Hellmann, M.D.; Ciuleanu, T.E.; Pluzanski, A.; Lee, J.S.; Otterson, G.A.; Audigier-Valette, C.; Minenza, E.; Linardou, H.; Burgers, S.; Salman, P.; et al. Nivolumab plus ipilimumab in lung cancer with a high tumor mutational burden. *N. Engl. J. Med.* **2018**, *378*, 2093–2104. [CrossRef]
50. Motzer, R.J.; Tannir, N.M.; McDermott, D.F.; Arén Frontera, O.; Melichar, B.; Choueiri, T.K.; Plimack, E.R.; Barthélémy, P.; Porta, C.; George, S.; et al. Nivolumab plus Ipilimumab versus Sunitinib in advanced renal-cell carcinoma. *N. Engl. J. Med.* **2018**, *378*, 1277–1290. [CrossRef]
51. Hodi, F.S.; Chiarion-Sileni, V.; Gonzalez, R.; Grob, J.J.; Rutkowski, P.; Cowey, C.L.; Lao, C.D.; Schadendorf, D.; Wagstaff, J.; Dummer, R.; et al. Nivolumab plus ipilimumab or nivolumab alone versus ipilimumab alone in advanced melanoma (CheckMate 067): 4-year outcomes of a multicentre, randomised, phase 3 trial. *Lancet Oncol.* **2018**, *19*, 1480–1492. [CrossRef]
52. Larkin, J.; Chiarion-Sileni, V.; Gonzalez, R.; Grob, J.J.; Rutkowski, P.; Lao, C.D.; Cowey, C.L.; Schadendorf, D.; Wagstaff, J.; Dummer, R.; et al. Five-year survival with combined nivolumab and ipilimumab in advanced melanoma. *N. Engl. J. Med.* **2019**, *381*, 1535–1546. [CrossRef] [PubMed]
53. Coppé, J.-P.; Desprez, P.-Y.; Krtolica, A.; Campisi, J. The Senescence-Associated Secretory Phenotype: The Dark Side of Tumor Suppression. *Annu. Rev. Pathol. Mech. Dis.* **2010**, *5*, 99–118. [CrossRef]
54. Rodier, F.; Coppé, J.P.; Patil, C.K.; Hoeijmakers, W.A.M.; Muñoz, D.P.; Raza, S.R.; Freund, A.; Campeau, E.; Davalos, A.R.; Campisi, J. Persistent DNA damage signalling triggers senescence-associated inflammatory cytokine secretion. *Nat. Cell Biol.* **2009**, *11*, 973–979. [CrossRef] [PubMed]
55. Mario Gonzalez-Meljem, J.; Haston, S.; Carreno, G.; Apps, J.R.; Pozzi, S.; Stache, C.; Kaushal, G.; Virasami, A.; Panousopoulos, L.; Neda Mousavy-Gharavy, S.; et al. Stem cell senescence drives age-attenuated induction of pituitary tumours in mouse models of paediatric craniopharyngioma. *Nat. Commun.* **2017**, *8*, 1819. [CrossRef]
56. Hickson, L.T.J.; Langhi Prata, L.G.P.; Bobart, S.A.; Evans, T.K.; Giorgadze, N.; Hashmi, S.K.; Herrmann, S.M.; Jensen, M.D.; Jia, Q.; Jordan, K.L.; et al. Senolytics decrease senescent cells in humans: Preliminary report from a clinical trial of Dasatinib plus Quercetin in individuals with diabetic kidney disease. *EBioMedicine* **2019**, *47*, 446–456. [CrossRef] [PubMed]
57. Ganau, L.; Prisco, L.; Ligarotti, G.K.I.; Ambu, R.; Ganau, M. Understanding the Pathological Basis of Neurological Diseases Through Diagnostic Platforms Based on Innovations in Biomedical Engineering: New Concepts and Theranostics Perspectives. *Medicines (Basel)* **2018**, *5*, 22. [CrossRef]
58. Ganau, M.; Paris, M.; Syrmos, N.; Ganau, L.; Ligarotti, G.K.I.; Moghaddamjou, A.; Prisco, L.; Ambu, R.; Chibbaro, S. How nanotechnology and biomedical engineering are supporting the identification of predictive biomarkers in neuro-oncology. *Medicines (Basel)* **2018**, *5*, 23. [CrossRef]

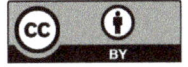

© 2020 by the authors. Licensee MDPI, Basel, Switzerland. This article is an open access article distributed under the terms and conditions of the Creative Commons Attribution (CC BY) license (http://creativecommons.org/licenses/by/4.0/).

MDPI
St. Alban-Anlage 66
4052 Basel
Switzerland
Tel. +41 61 683 77 34
Fax +41 61 302 89 18
www.mdpi.com

Journal of Clinical Medicine Editorial Office
E-mail: jcm@mdpi.com
www.mdpi.com/journal/jcm

www.ingramcontent.com/pod-product-compliance
Lightning Source LLC
LaVergne TN
LVHW070541100526
838202LV00012B/348